Growing Up Cavity Free

About the Author

Stephen J. Moss, DDS, MS, practiced pediatric dentistry in Manhattan for more than 30 years. He serves as Chairman and Professor of the Department of Pediatric Dentistry at the New York University College of Dentistry and was recently appointed Division Head of Growth and Developmental Sciences in recognition of his abilities in early and interceptive orthodontics. Dr Moss is a diplomate and past president of the American Academy of Pediatric Dentistry, has served on the Advisory Committee to the National Caries Program of the National Institute of Dental Research, and has been quoted regularly as a spokesperson for the American Dental Association. A foremost authority on dentistry for children, he has appeared on "The Today Show," "Good Morning America," "CNN World News," and "Sesame Street," and is a consultant for many consumer magazines. Dr Moss is known worldwide as a lecturer devoted to educating health professionals, parents, and future pediatric dentists.

Growing Up Cavity Free

A Parent's Guide to Prevention

Stephen J. Moss, DDS, MS

quintessence
books

Quintessence Publishing Co, Inc
Chicago, Berlin, London, Tokyo,
Moscow, Prague, Sophia, Warsaw

Library of Congress Cataloging-in-Publication Data

Moss, Stephen J.
  Growing up cavity free: a parent's guide to prevention / Stephen J. Moss.
    p.   cm.
  Includes index.
  ISBN 0-86715-256-7
  1. Teeth—Care and hygiene.   2. Children—Dental care.   I. Title.
RK61.M869   1993
617.6'01—dc20   93-8190
                                                                       CIP

© 1993 by Quintessence Publishing Co, Inc, Carol Stream, Illinois.
All rights reserved.

Cover Photography: Ronald Cecconi
Editor: Lori A. Bateman
Designer and Production: Jennifer A. Sabella

Composition: Focus Graphics, St Louis, MO
Printing and Binding: Federated Printing, Providence, RI

To my father
Dr Hyman H. Moss

Few things disturbed my father as much as when a youngster's first visit to his office was made as a result of a toothache. He believed such an initiation might scar the child for life and that he or she would forever mistakenly associate dentists with fear and discomfort.

When he read my first book, *Your Child's Teeth*, he exclaimed, "How marvelous growing up cavity free . . . if only it could become a reality." Dedicated to his memory, and his desire to see a generation of cavity-free children, this book is a reflection of his concern for others, his kindness, and most of all, his love of children.

Contents

Introduction 1

1. Your Child's Teeth Before Birth and During Infancy 5
The Developing Tooth 5
What to Do Before the Baby Comes: Eat Right 6
The New Baby's Mouth at Birth 8
What You Can Do Before Teeth Come in 10
Pacifiers and Sucking Habits 12
How Nursing Affects Your Baby's Teeth and Jaws 14
Cleaning Routine for Infants 18
The Good Effects of Early Chewing Habits 20
Mouth Infections 21
Tongue Tie 22
Children With Special Needs 22

**2. Your Child's Teeth From Babyhood Through
   Adolescence 25**
When Do the First Teeth Appear? 25
Teething 30

Those Important Primary Teeth **32**
Cleaning the First Teeth **38**
Sealants: Long-Lasting Dental "Insurance" **41**
Tooth Position and Bad Habits **42**
Speech and Teeth **48**
Cleaning Techniques as Your Child Grows Older **49**
Green, Black, Orange Stains **52**
The Most Important Teeth: The 6-Year Molars **55**
What to Do About a Loose Primary Tooth:
 Just Pull It Out! **55**
Injuries and Traumas **56**
Protecting Your Child's Teeth at School and at Play **62**
Teeth and Teenagers **63**
Report Card—3 Years **67**
Report Card—6 Years **68**
Report Card—9 Years **69**
Report Card—12 Years **70**

3. **The Amazing Tooth** **71**
How a Tooth Begins **71**
The Parts of a Tooth **72**
What a Tooth is Made of **72**
The Environment of the Teeth **76**

4. **A Complete Guide to Clean Teeth** **81**
Tipping the Scale Toward No Decay **81**
What is Plaque? **82**
Plaque Control **85**
How to Protect the Tooth's Surface From Decay **94**

5. **The Fluoride Story** **97**
Questions Commonly Asked About Fluoride **97**
Filling Your Child's Fluoride Reservoir **103**
A Multiple Approach **107**

6. **Diet and Dental Health** **109**
You Are What You Eat, But . . . **109**
Food and Tooth Decay **110**
Leisurely Dining, Bacteria Style **110**
The Bottom Line: Diet Is Only Part of the Puzzle **112**

7. **A Visit to the Dentist** **115**
Choosing a Dentist **115**

Evaluating a Dentist **117**
How to Help Your Child Have a Pleasant Experience
  at the Dentist's Office **118**
Getting Ready for a Visit **119**
Should You Accompany Your Child Into the
  Treatment Room? **121**
How Often Should You Visit the Dentist? **124**
X-ray Examinations **124**
Anesthesia **125**

8. **All About Orthodontics 127**
When is Orthodontics Needed? **127**
Occlusion **128**
Malocclusion **129**
Preventive Orthodontics **129**
How Orthodontics Works **132**
How Long Will It Take? **134**
How Much Will It Cost? **134**
How Much Will It Hurt? **135**
Removable or Fixed Appliances? **135**
Oral Hygiene During Orthodontics **136**

9. **Preventing Dental Problems: Past, Present, Future 137**
Background of the Preventive Dentistry Movement **137**
The Numbers Game **139**
Dentistry of the Future **140**
Conclusion **142**

Acknowledgments

My sincerest gratitude is extended to:

My wife, Lydia, for maintaining an atmosphere of love and tranquility, enabling me to work pressure free.

My sons, Jonathan and David, for remaining cavity free into their mid-20s, proving that prevention works.

Dr Haim Sarnat, chairman and professor of the Department of Pediatric Dentistry at Tel Aviv University, Israel, for graciously reading my manuscript and making numerous worthwhile and important suggestions.

Dr Lorraine Arav, a talented pediatric dentist in Paris, France, for her research and creative suggestions dealing with caries, diet, and infant care.

Dr Gary Goldstein, Dr Mladen Kuftinec, Dr Linda Rosenberg, and Dr Neal Herman, for collecting and editing the illustrative photographs.

The staff and faculty of the Department of Pediatric Dentistry at the New York University College of Dentistry, for the loyalty and support that enabled me to gain the experience necessary to create this work.

The American Academy of Pediatric Dentistry, for the opportunity to work with them to promote pediatric dentistry and the lifetime benefits of pediatric dental care.

Introduction

In 1977 I wrote a book, *Your Child's Teeth*, intended to give parents the most up-to-date advice on how to rear dentally healthy children. At that time, I proposed a simple idea: we can break the chain of tooth decay.

Much has changed in the years since. Dentistry for children is, after all, based on science, and scientific advancement in this field has been remarkable. In fact, we've learned so much in the last decade or so that I find it necessary to rewrite and update my book.

But one thing hasn't changed. I and my colleagues believe more strongly than ever that dental disease is totally preventable. Your children can have strong, straight, sound teeth, and it's much more easily accomplished than you may think.

How, you may wonder, can I be so sure about that? Consider this: among the general population, half of American youngsters under age 12 have no cavities; yet if we look at just the families of pediatric dentists, *9 out of 10 of the children under age 12 have no cavities*.

If that suggests to you that pediatric dentists might be on to a good thing, you're right. But the secrets of our success are simple things that anyone can live with. In other words, don't look here for complicated formulas, rigid rules, and time-consuming regimens that will place yet another burden on your already busy lives.

As I said in my first book, bad teeth don't "run in the family." There is just no hereditary excuse for cavities or for crooked teeth. What pass from one generation to the next are customs, lifestyles, and attitudes toward oral cleanliness. Armed with the right information and intentions, you can give your own children a foundation of good dental health that you yourself may have lacked.

As proof, I offer my own family. Both my wife and I experienced a sad history of dental decay, despite the facts that my father was a dentist and that my wife's family could have afforded the best dental care available. We decided to try to give our children a better start.

Today, our sons Jonathan and David are in their mid-20s. Both have strong, straight, cavity-free teeth—the sort that my wife and I missed out on. Our family's experience is evidence that bad teeth are not inherited, and cavities are not inevitable.

To prove it for yourself, read on.

My Family Album: How Defensive Dentistry Works

Both my wife and I have had many cavities. We have spent hours having them repaired. We must have imparted some susceptibility to our two sons. Yet by practicing defensive dentistry in our home, we have overcome the children's susceptibility to cavities. As you can see from these photographs, we have given them perfect teeth. You can do this for your children.

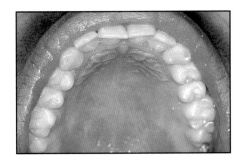

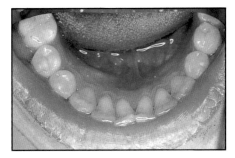

Jonathan, age 27

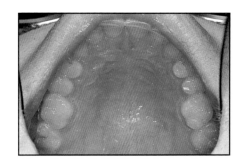

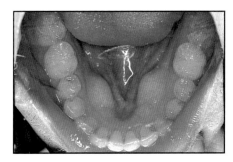

David, age 25

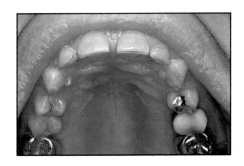

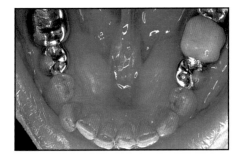

My teeth

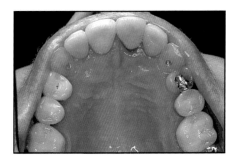

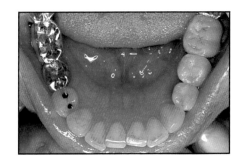

My wife's teeth

Your Child's Teeth Before Birth and During Infancy

The Developing Tooth

About 3 months after conception your baby's teeth are already beginning to form and to be recognizable. Which teeth form before birth? Some parts of all of the 20 primary teeth. (Primary teeth also go by the names baby teeth, milk teeth, and first teeth.) Except for a tiny piece of the first permanent molar, the rest of the permanent teeth begin forming right after birth.

If the baby is going to be a thumb sucker, chances are the habit is already well underway by the seventh month in the uterus. (Knowing that today most dentists and doctors believe that thumb suckers are born, not made, may help you to relax later.) In the weeks before birth, the baby is already making sucking and chewing movements in preparation for nursing. In short, even before birth, the mouth is getting ready for its complex tasks.

A nutritious, balanced diet is good for anyone, anytime. But for an expectant mother, it pays double benefits by contributing to the health of both mother and child. However, with the exception of maintaining a balanced diet,

Although the first teeth will not make their appearance in the baby's mouth until about 6 months after birth, the primary teeth begin to form as early as the seventh week of pregnancy. This is the developmental pattern:

Tooth-bud formation
↓
Beginning of crown formation
↓
Completion of crown
↓
Beginning of root formation
↓
Eruption of tooth into mouth
↓
Completion of root formation

True or False?

"The baby took all the calcium from my teeth!"

False. If the mother has sufficient calcium in her diet, there's no problem. If her diet is deficient in calcium, the calcium requirements of the embryo will be met first, and some of the calcium may come from the mother's bones; it will not come from her teeth.

There are hormonal changes during pregnancy, and one of the results of these changes is swelling of the gums. Swollen gums harbor food debris and bacteria; gum disease and decay may develop. You might blame your toothache on pregnancy, but don't blame your baby. Just be especially careful. Brush. Floss. Get a thorough cleaning from a dentist. But avoid having x-rays taken, if possible.

staying well, and avoiding harmful drugs, there is really not much a mother-to-be can do to affect her baby's teeth directly. Most of what goes on in the embryonic stages takes place automatically. The calcium, phosphorus, and other minerals that are needed to form a baby's developing teeth are taken from the mother's bloodstream, and unless she is actually undernourished, nothing will interfere with the ability of the baby's tooth-forming cells to turn these basic minerals into normal dentin and enamel cells.

If a child is going to get cavities (or *caries*) in the first set of teeth, it will probably be in one of two areas: the biting surfaces of the molars, or between the molars, where two teeth come into contact with each other.

Why talk about this now? Because now—before birth— is when the top surfaces and the side surfaces of the molar teeth are beginning to form. How resistant these caries-sensitive surfaces will be depends on how well they mineralize. The mother, by balancing the necessary calcium, phosphorus, and vitamins in her bloodstream, contributes to successful tooth development.

We know that fluoride is a great help to developing teeth, but not much fluoride gets into them. Because there is no way to get more fluoride into an unborn baby's teeth through the mother's diet, strengthening the teeth with fluoride will have to wait until later.

What To Do Before the Baby Comes: Eat Right

For 9 months before birth, the baby depends entirely on his or her mother for nourishment. This nourishment comes from two sources: the food the mother eats and the tissues of her body. The calcium, phosphorus, and vitamins needed for good teeth and bones, for instance, can be supplied in a balanced diet that contains four basic food groups. A pregnant woman should eat a variety of (1) dairy products; (2) meat, poultry, and fish; (3) fruits and vegetables; and (4) enriched or whole-grain cereals and breads.

The menu provided here will give the expectant mother an idea of how to plan her diet to supply the nutrients she needs; her obstetrician can also provide helpful nutritional suggestions and answer specific questions about diet and weight during pregnancy. If the doctor advises that a vitamin-mineral supplement be taken, it should be regarded as extra insurance—not as a substitute for good nutrition.

Suggested Menu for Pregnant Women*

BREAKFAST *(choose one from each category)*

Choice of: Orange juice
            Orange
            Grapefruit half
Choice of: One egg, boiled or poached
            Bran cereal and milk
            Whole grain cereal and milk
Choice of: Buttered toast (one slice)
            Muffin
            One glass of milk

LUNCH *(choose one from each category)*

Choice of: Melon
            Fresh fruit salad
            Fresh vegetable salad
Choice of: Chicken
            Cottage Cheese
            Fish (if canned tuna, eat only waterpacked)

MIDAFTERNOON SNACK *(choose one)*

Choice of: Fresh fruit/cheese and crackers

DINNER *(choose one from each category)*

Choice of: Meat
            Chicken
            Fish (broiled, baked, poached, or boiled)
            Seafood
Choice of: Two green or yellow vegetables
            Tossed salad, one vegetable
Choice of: Bread or roll
            Baked or boiled potato or rice
            Small portion of pasta

*From *The Doctor's Guide to Pregnancy After 30*, by Ronald M. Caplan, MD. Used with permission.

Three Things That May Happen to the Expectant Mother
That Could Directly Affect Her Baby's Teeth

1. If the mother gets a fever from a virus or some other infection (a common occurrence between the fifth and ninth months of pregnancy), the delicate balance of calcium and phosphorous salts in her bloodstream could be upset. This would affect the quality and quantity of tooth structure that is forming in the fetus. The disruption in tooth structure formation will continue for as long as it takes the mother's system to regain its balance.

2. If the mother's physician gives her an antibiotic containing tetracycline, the developing fetal teeth might become stained. Later, when the teeth come into the mouth, they will be discolored. The color may range from dark gray through yellow to bright orange, depending on how much tetracycline the mother gets, how long she takes it, and at what time during pregnancy. Most physicians don't prescribe tetracycline for pregnant mothers; its use is becoming rare. Nevertheless, a woman who is pregnant but doesn't yet "show" should tell any healthcare provider—general physician, dentist (because of x-ray and antibiotic risks), even chiropractor—that she's expecting.

3. If the expectant mother gives birth before term, it is possible that the child's teeth will be affected. There is some evidence today that full-term children have fewer cavities. This is because those areas of the teeth that are mineralizing just around the time of birth are the ones most susceptible to decay.

The New Baby's Mouth at Birth

At birth, your baby's health care starts with a thorough examination by the obstetrician and the pediatrician. Any congenital abnormalities in the dentition, such as a cleft lip or palate, should be diagnosed by these doctors and the baby should be referred for proper treatment. But remember that unusual and rare conditions are just that—unusual and rare. Your baby will probably have the good start in life for which every parent hopes. If there is a problem that necessitates surgery, my advice is to wait as long as possible, unless the problem interferes with the baby's ability to eat and survive. It's tough on the parents psychologically, but the older the child is before subjected to surgery, the bigger the parts that the surgeon will have to work with—and the final result will be better for the child.

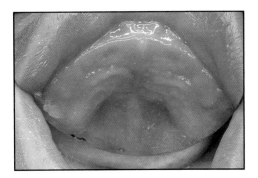

Mouth of the newborn. Notice the gum pads and "Epstein's pearls" (little white spots on the roof of the mouth, generally disappear within 10 to 14 days).

Epstein's Pearls

Sometimes, shortly after birth, parents or physicians notice little white spots on the upper palate (the roof of the mouth). These are little keratinized structures called "Epstein's pearls." (Keratin is a tough, fibrous protein found in nails, hair, and teeth.) They are not significant and will disappear within 10 to 14 days.

Babies Born With a Tooth in the Mouth

Some babies are born with teeth in their mouth. The teeth may be apparent immediately or may appear 1 or 2 days after birth. Usually these are not extra teeth; they are primary teeth that are forming close to the mucosa. If the baby is healthy and the teeth do not interfere with nursing or cause lesions on the tongue, they should be left in place. There is no reason to fear that the tooth will be aspirated (inhaled) by a healthy child with all his or her protective mechanisms.

Eruption Cysts

Later, small cysts may develop on the gum pads. These are the sacs that surround a developing tooth. They are called "eruption cysts" and tend to disappear after a few days. Don't let anyone cut or puncture them. They have poor circulation and can easily become infected.

What You Can Do Before Teeth Come in

Immediately after your baby's birth, you as parents can start to do something about your child's teeth. What you do during the first months will set the stage for what happens to your baby's teeth for the rest of his or her life. It's not too early to think about the permanent teeth, which are developing in the baby's jaw while you are waiting for the first primary tooth to erupt.

I firmly believe that the most important thing you as parents can do to ensure your baby's oral health is to mind your own oral hygiene. Babies aren't born with a mouthful of cavity-causing bacteria; they acquire the interlopers after birth. And where do the bacteria come from? Recent research clearly indicates that oral bacteria are transferred from parent to baby during normal cuddling, kissing, and play.

Fortunately, cavity-causing microorganisms do not colonize easily in the infant's mouth. Before bacteria can take hold, it must be reintroduced repeatedly, every couple of hours for a few days. So for baby's sake as well as yours, do all you can to control the microorganisms in your own mouth. That is, get into the habit of brushing twice a day, flossing, and seeing your dentist for regular checkups. You'll make the perfect dental role model, to boot.

That's not all you can do to help baby avoid cavities. Statistics indicate that if your child is going to get a cavity in the primary teeth, it will most probably be on the biting surface or side of the first primary molar. These are the very areas that are developing during the first 3 years of life. If your child is going to get a cavity in the permanent teeth, the story is exactly the same—the biting surface and side are the most vulnerable, and they, too, begin mineralizing from birth on. Try to think of these areas as especially cavity prone. The best method of protecting them is to get fluoride into them.

... the most important thing you as parents can do to ensure your baby's oral health is to mind your own oral hygiene.

Fluoride for Infants

One of the best ways to help developing teeth form perfectly and make them resistant to decay is to expose them early to fluoride. Fluoride has been so effective in helping prevent cavities in children that some scientists are beginning to call dental caries a fluoride-deficiency disease. Fluoride, a naturally occurring substance, becomes incorporated into the developing tooth enamel, making it 50% to 80% less susceptible to decay.

So if babies knew what was good for them, they'd howl for fluoride. "No problem," say the parents, "our community's water supply is fluoridated." Fine, but if a mother is breast feeding and not giving her baby a supplemental bottle, the baby is probably not getting any fluoride. Even when the mother drinks fluoridated water, her milk contains almost no fluoride. Breast-fed babies should receive supplementary fluoride until they are weaned. If your baby is bottle-fed, it's also a good idea to ask your dentist or physician if a fluoride-vitamin supplement is needed.

It was once assumed that infants living in communities with nonfluoridated drinking water would probably receive only a small amount of fluoride each day. However, recent research suggests that even in these areas infants are receiving more dietary fluoride than was previously thought. "Hidden" sources such as commercially prepared concentrated liquid formulas and reconstituted juices often contain fluoride. The amount varies among products, even those produced by the same manufacturer, because the products may be made in different cities.

If your baby's physician or dentist advises a liquid fluoride-vitamin supplement, ask for one in which the full dose is delivered in a fairly large quantity—about 4 milliliters. A more concentrated supplement may require only one or two tiny drops of liquid (1 milliliter) per dose. It's too easy for an extra drop or two to fall into the baby's mouth, and that can lead to overdosage. When it comes to fluoride supplementation, more is not better. This is a case where a little is best.

. . . if a mother is breast feeding and not giving her baby a supplemental bottle, the baby is probably not getting any fluoride.

Well Baby = Healthy Teeth

Try to keep your baby well. Of course, you'd do this anyway, but there's an important connection between general health and teeth. An infectious illness or a high fever affects the adjustment of calcium and phosphorous salts in the baby's bloodstream. This means that the primary and permanent teeth developing at this time will mineralize imperfectly, making them more susceptible to cavities.

If you've been thinking that certain childhood diseases are inevitable and that it's best to "go ahead and get them over with," then it's time to change your mind. Prevent childhood diseases until your child is 3½ or 4 years old. Give your child's permanent front teeth a chance to form.

• Try to avoid giving your baby the antibiotic tetracycline or its derivatives. Today there are good alternative antibiotics. Tetracycline, especially during the first year of life, will stain primary and permanent teeth.

• Keep a record of childhood illnesses. If your baby is ill during the first year, before the first tooth erupts into the mouth, special care will have to be taken to keep the baby's mouth clean. The teeth may come into the mouth looking fine to the mother and father—and even to the dentist. But because of imperfect mineralization, these teeth may have a built-in susceptibility to cavities. When your child goes to the dentist for the first time, make a point of giving your dentist information about childhood illnesses, so that it becomes part of your child's record.

Pacifiers and Sucking Habits

Pacifiers come in all shapes and sizes. The thumb and the fingers are the ones that nature provides; the rubber and plastic models from the drugstore are provided by Mom and Dad.

Right from birth—and even before—most babies have an urge to suck on anything that is placed in or near the mouth. This is an inborn, natural reflex and should not be discouraged. Many babies get enough sucking by nursing or using a bottle with a proper nipple (that is, a non-free-flowing type). Other babies seem to need more of this activity.

Research to date indicates that children should be encouraged to work the muscles in their tongue and cheeks, and to exercise the swallowing reflex as much and as soon as possible, in order to get their muscles into proper balance and thus develop a musculature that will lead the teeth into the mouth in a straight, even position. Further, the child who sucks vigorously and is given an opportunity to practice chewing is preparing a good environment for the primary teeth to erupt into. Teeth don't know where they're going—there's no game plan. Have you ever seen, in the bottom front teeth of an older child, the permanent tooth that comes in behind the front primary tooth? The tongue begins to push that tooth forward, the lips hold it back, and the dynamics of the mouth enable it to go where it's needed.

Children should be encouraged to chew and bite as soon as possible—even before the first tooth comes into the mouth. For many children, teething rings and toys and natural foods can serve this purpose. If your child uses a pacifier, don't worry. If your child doesn't lose interest in the pacifier before the permanent incisors erupt, *then* begin to worry (and see Chapter 2 for the discussion of tooth position and bad habits). The only advantage of an artificial over a natural pacifier (thumb, fingers) is that it is likely to be lost, and at some future date the habit will more easily be given up. How forceful the parents can be at that time without disturbing their relationship with the child and with each other is an important consideration. Try to evaluate the problem on a rational basis.

The effect that the pacifier habit will have on teeth is usually proportional to the amount of time the child has worked at the habit. Accordingly, 3 hours a day is better than 5 hours, 2 years is better than 3 years, and this, in turn, is better than allowing the child to continue the habit into the fourth or fifth year. If a child can be encouraged to work at it less and less each day, there will be fewer problems later. One way to do this would be to make a habit of removing the pacifier or thumb from the child's mouth once he or she has fallen asleep.

Of all malocclusions (improperly positioned teeth) that occur, those caused solely by thumb sucking or pacifiers are the easiest to correct. But if you'd rather avoid them now than correct them later, remember the following guidelines on sucking habits.

Safe Use of Pacifiers

- **NEVER** *tie a pacifier around a baby's neck. Between 1985 and 1990, the US Consumer Product Safety Commission received reports of 21 strangulation deaths that involved pacifiers tied around a child's neck.*
- *Look for a pacifier with sturdy, one-piece construction, made of nontoxic, flexible material, with an easily grasped handle.*
- *The pacifier should have a shield or mouthguard that can't be separated from the nipple, has two ventilating holes, and is too large to be swallowed.*
- *The nipple should be intact, with no holes or tears, so that a piece can't break off in the baby's mouth. Parents should pull on the nipple to test it, and replace the pacifier when the nipple shows signs of wear.*

Courtesy of Dr Arthur J. Nowak.

Guidelines on Sucking Habits

- All children need to suck and bite. But when such activity is carried on for prolonged periods of time, it becomes a pernicious habit. The earlier it is stopped (preferably by the time the child is 4½ years old), the less damage it will do. Damage to the teeth is a function of time. The longer the child retains the habit, the greater the chance for improperly positioned teeth to develop.

- However, until the permanent teeth erupt, it's really not worth hassling your child and aggravating yourself in an attempt to break a sucking habit. If the habit is still present when the permanent teeth start to erupt, you will either have to stop the habit (see Chapter 2) or resign yourself to the probability of having to correct misaligned teeth.

Often a dentist examining a child for the first time will count the child's fingers before looking at the teeth. This allows the dentist to make body contact gradually, and in a nonthreatening area of the body. It gets the child's attention. And it gives the dentist information. When the dentist sees an exceptionally clean thumb or finger, he or she knows the child has a built-in pacifier.

Children with a strong, persistent urge to suck will sometimes substitute other activities as they grow older. See the section on bad habits (pages 42-48) for a fuller discussion.

How Nursing Affects Your Baby's Teeth and Jaws

One of the purposes of the baby's nursing (besides the obvious one of obtaining nourishment) is to educate the muscles of the lips, cheeks, tongue, and jaw to more and more mature ways of handling fuel for the body. These muscles, along with taste buds, heat-sensitive nerve endings, and salivary glands (and later the teeth), make up the mouth's apparatus for evaluating, manipulating, chewing, and swallowing food.

Nursing affects the development of muscular patterns. If an unnatural pattern is formed, . . . the child may develop a malocclusion.

Nursing affects the development of muscular patterns. If an unnatural pattern is formed, the erupting teeth will not be directed by the muscles into the proper position, and the child may develop a malocclusion.

Differences Between Breast Feeding and Bottle Feeding

The breast-fed child must work the tongue and the muscles around the mouth vigorously, in a pattern perfected throughout the evolutionary process. It's an activity requiring a great deal of skill. In addition, the child nursing from the breast is generally held upright—the natural position— with gravity working correctly on the muscles associated with swallowing. A mother may decide to breast feed her child until all the front primary teeth are in, at about the age of 2. Once the primary teeth are in, the tongue adapts to the shape of the teeth, the swallowing pattern changes, and the child is ready to move on to new foods.

When babies nurse from a breast substitute — a nipple on a bottle, that is — the action is entirely different. Milk is not supplied on demand but often flows from the bottle in a continuous stream, and the muscles of the mouth don't have to work as hard. Babies nursing while lying on their backs must keep their tongue in an unnatural forward position to keep from drowning!

If you breast feed for a while and then wean the baby to a bottle and not to a cup, observe the tips at the bottom of this page. Bad habits start as early as birth and can be initiated any time thereafter.

Baby-Bottle Tooth Decay

What's the worst thing you can do to brand-new babies?
1. Forget their vitamins.
2. Drop them on their head.
3. Put them in their crib with a bottle at nap time or let them walk around during the day with a bottle in their mouth.

A dentist would choose number 3. Tooth decay is practically epidemic among children who have been allowed to use a bottle — or breast — as a pacifier. (The photographs on the following page illustrate the danger.)

Baby-bottle tooth decay, the most common reason for tooth decay before age 3, is caused by a combination of factors: (1) failing to clean both baby's *and parents'* mouths daily and (2) using the feeding bottle as a pacifier.

Important Tips on Bottle Feeding

1. Encourage your baby to stay in an upright position while nursing with a bottle.
2. Use a bottle with a nipple that has a small hole. Check to see that the baby is required to work to get milk from the bottle. There are several types of nipples on the market. Find one that is non-free-flowing and makes the child move the cheeks, tongue, and jaws. Many orthodontic problems in young children may be caused by an imbalance in musculature.
3. Introduce the child to drinking from a cup as soon as possible.
4. Let the baby feed from the bottle at intervals, as though it were a breast.
5. Day or night, never use a nursing bottle as a pacifier. Milk or juice that constantly bathes the teeth can lead to severe cavities.
6. Most important of all, clean the mouth and teeth twice a day — after breakfast and before bed at night.

The Danger of Using a Nursing Bottle as a Pacifier

The upper front teeth of these two preschool children show the destruction that can occur when a child whose teeth have not been cleaned is allowed to sleep with a bottle or walk around with it during the day.

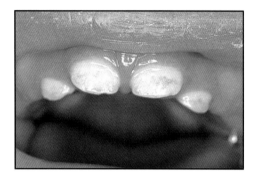

Tommy is only 18 months of age and is already showing the first signs of baby-bottle tooth decay.

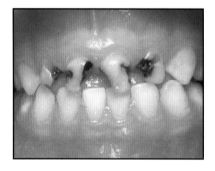

Cindy, age 3, used the bottle as a pacifier until past her second birthday.

If a child is pacified or put to bed with a bottle of milk or juice, the child's mouth is continually bathed with the liquid. When the teeth have not been properly cleaned, this situation offers a virtual feast to the decay-causing bacteria that are on the child's teeth. Although cavities may not appear until the fourth or fifth year of life, they can be the result of sleeping with a nursing bottle for long periods of time. Even breast-fed infants, if they have dirty teeth and fall asleep nursing, are prime candidates for baby-bottle tooth decay.

Typically, decay affects all the upper teeth and sometimes the lower back teeth, but almost never the lower front teeth. In part, that's because when the child is nursing, the tongue covers and protects the lower teeth while the nipple is pressed between the top surface of the tongue and the upper jaw. Also, while the child nurses, saliva tends to pool around the lower front teeth, continually cleansing them. Dentistry is just beginning to appreciate the important role saliva plays in dental health (see Chapter 3).

If a nursing bottle is still being used when the baby's teeth begin to appear, it should be given only for short periods of time, when the baby is awake and sitting up. If using a bottle for a pacifier, put plain water in the bottle. Water is harmless to teeth and, if the local water supply is fluoridated, may even be beneficial.

Unprepared as you may be for it, decay can actually start in primary teeth soon after they erupt.

If a child aged 2 or younger comes into my office with cavities, I know before he or she even sits in my chair that one or more of the above practices has not been followed.

We can see from statistics the effect that the bottle habit can have on the incidence of decay in primary teeth. The average 3- to 4-year-old has had to have one to two-and-a-half decayed teeth filled. A child whose dental deterioration traces back to no oral hygiene and many hours spent with juice or formula bathing the teeth can expect to have more than 10 decayed teeth filled in the primary set. When your child grows beyond the bottle-feeding age, get rid of the bottle.

Follow These Practices—They Decrease Your Infant's Risk of Tooth Decay

- Clean your infant's teeth twice daily.

- Keep your own teeth scrupulously clean while your infant's teeth are erupting.

- Do not permit your child to use a bottle containing milk, juice, or anything other than plain water as a daytime or nighttime pacifier.

- After your child has learned to drink from a cup, do not give him or her a bottle containing juice or sweetened liquid throughout the day.

- Do not give your baby a pacifier dipped in honey, jelly, or sugar. If such an outrageous impulse occurs to you, squelch it!

Cleaning Routine for Infants

If we could get rid of plaque, most of our problems would be over. But as long as we harbor bacteria in our mouths (and we do), and as long as we continue to put food into our mouths (and we will), we're going to have plaque.

Plaque is an almost invisible film containing a sticky substance that coats the teeth and sets the stage for dental decay and gum disease. The oral bacteria that live in plaque, reacting with various food residues, excrete an acid that, held to the tooth in the sticky film, goes to work to break down the tooth structure. Plaque must be carefully removed every day from the mouth of anyone who intends to have healthy teeth and gums. *Regular cleaning should begin even before your child's teeth have erupted.*

The gum pads in your child's mouth are covered with the same tissue that covers newly erupted teeth. The colonies of bacteria that form on the gum pads are the same as those that form on the erupting teeth. By keeping the gum pads

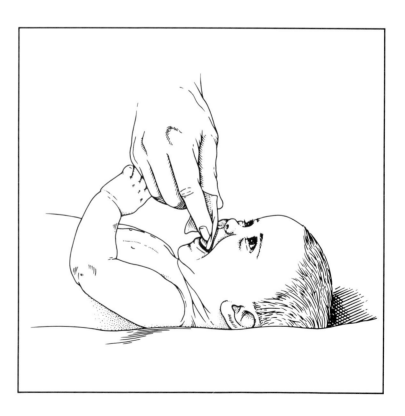

The easiest way to clean the mouths of infants is to lay them down with their head in your lap, feet pointing away. A small piece of gauze can be used.

How to Clean an Infant's Mouth

1. The easiest way to carry out this cleaning procedure is to lay the baby down with the head in your lap and feet pointing away.

2. To open the baby's mouth, you may need to slide your forefinger along the inside of the baby's cheek and press down on the back part of the lower gum pad.

3. Take a piece of gauze (2 inches x 2 inches) between your thumb and forefinger and wipe vigorously over the ridge of the baby's top and bottom jaws. Use only the tiniest dab of fluoride toothpaste on the gauze and try to ensure that the baby doesn't swallow toothpaste. (As an alternative to gauze, there are many new oral-hygiene products available today designed specifically for infants. These include wipes, brushes, and finger cots, as well as toothpastes that taste good to babies and don't foam or create a "burning" sensation on tender infant tissues.)

4. Use just enough pressure to remove the film that is covering the child's teeth and gum pads. Think of the action of your fingers as being the same as squeezing a marshmallow. There is some evidence that this kind of cleaning routine can help reduce teething pain.

5. Clean your baby's mouth this way twice a day—after breakfast and after the last meal in the evening. It should take about 2 minutes.

clean, you can remove food residues. You can also reduce the oral bacteria and cut down on the acid produced.

With less acid in the mouth, the baby will have an easier time teething; with a lower bacteria count, the baby may even have fewer colds during the first year. And the baby's first teeth will arrive in a clean, plaque-free environment.

The simple steps involved in cleaning an infant's mouth are part of the foundation of early prevention. It is the parents' responsibility, because children can no more do it than they can clean their ears or trim their nails. And yet, simple as it is, it involves a complex behavioral change on the part of parents, because it means adding a habit to your life that was not part of your own growing up and that is probably not observed by your peers.

Many parents are afraid to look into a child's mouth; they regard the mouth as part of the inside of the body and, therefore, somehow inaccessible. They have no cultural basis for such a procedure. (Their friends don't do it; their parents didn't do it.) And they fear they are going to introduce some infection. (Did you ever try to make a list of the things that go in and out of a baby's mouth every day? A clean piece of gauze on a parent's finger is nothing!)

The first time you clean your child's mouth, you may notice a tiny bit of bleeding from the gums. This doesn't mean you're pushing too hard; it means the gum tissue was already irritated. Keep at it for a few days—the condition will clear up.

It may take some effort on your part to get as interested in cleaning the mouth as you are in cleaning and caring for other parts of the child's body. But, although the baby may object initially, parents who have adopted the routine find that the child begins to enjoy it and that it can be done rapidly and effectively.

The Good Effects of Early Chewing Habits

What did babies eat before there were formulas and pabulum and baby foods?

For thousands of years, children began to eat available, natural foods about the time they gave up nursing. Hard to believe, isn't it?

Children can be encouraged to get into the habit of chewing before any teeth erupt into their mouths. The gum pads provide children with strong biting surfaces. They serve the same purpose as the toothless ridges in a 60-year-old person who goes on enjoying a varied diet. Children can chew food without teeth.

Healthy children have amazing reflexes that will prevent them from swallowing food they cannot handle. As soon as children are able to grasp food, they should be encouraged to chew it. The tougher the food, the harder its consistency, the better it will be for the child. Be sensible, of course. Don't give your child small, hard foods like peanuts or other items that might cause choking.

Lazy chewing habits cause cavities and—this may surprise you—malocclusion (improper occlusion, or bite). Possibly one of the causes of orthodontic problems is that children are kept on soft foods for such long periods of time, just when their muscles and neuromuscular pathways are developing.

Just as many child psychologists believe that personality traits develop when children are young, many pediatric

Possibly one of the causes of orthodontic problems is that children are kept on soft foods for such long periods of time, just when their muscles and neuromuscular pathways are developing.

dentists think that preferences for soft foods (which will not naturally clean the teeth and will cause more cavities) and lazy chewing habits (which will lead to crooked teeth) are developed with the solicitous help of attentive parents who mistakenly weed out hard foods and feed their children soft foods—sometimes even after the children are 12 months old.

Fortunately, the trend today is to start babies on solid foods at about 6 months of age and quickly progress to feeding real table food. If you are willing to try, you will find that children as young as 7 or 8 months can and will chew when given the chance. Try introducing to the baby's diet such challenging foods as carrot shavings, celery strips, chewy toast, as well as crisp apple bits and pear slices.

Mouth Infections

As you become more familiar with the geography of your baby's mouth, you'll be quicker to notice anything unusual going on there. In general, the mouth has great resistance to infection. If the baby does get an infection of the mouth, it will usually be either cold sores or thrush. Both infections are often associated with high fever.

Thrush

Thrush (moniliasis) is recognized by white patches on the tongue and lips; it should be treated with antibiotics.

Cold Sores

Cold sores (herpes stomatitis) generally develop around the lips and inside the mouth and often look like little bubbles at first. The lesions usually last 8 to 10 days. There is no medicine that will help shorten the period of time that they will last, so a philosophical attitude is recommended. Don't give your child spicy or acidic foods, such as orange juice, and avoid mouthwashes. You can provide a little short-term relief if there are small, isolated lesions on cheeks and lips: dry them and place small dabs of petroleum jelly on them.

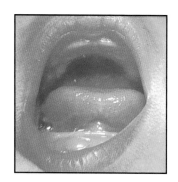

Tongue tie of the newborn. After a few months, the tissue at the bottom of the tongue will disappear.

Tongue Tie

At birth, and for a few days after, the mouth contains a little membrane that "ties" the tongue to the gum just behind the lower arch. This membrane places the tongue in the proper position for the child to nurse; during nursing the nipple is compressed between the upper gum pad and the top of the tongue. The membrane usually disappears in a few days and the child is able to stretch the tongue forward.

In some instances, the membrane turns into heavy tissue and the tip of the tongue is locked into position and cannot be extended. This condition has been known to cause problems with the position of erupting teeth.

When your child is about 4 months of age, try this simple test: see if your child is able stick the tip of the tongue out of the mouth in the direction of the nose. How? Try making faces, encouraging the child to imitate you. If it appears that there is a problem, report it to your dentist.

Children With Special Needs

Some children may be said to have a dental disability. The condition may have existed since birth—a cleft palate, for instance—or may develop later. Massive cavities due to poor hygiene or baby-bottle tooth decay fall into the second category. So do trauma disabilities, such as broken and injured teeth. Still other children may have mental or physical problems that make them unable to cope with ordinary dental home care.

Just as the parents and child adapt to the demands of a

special condition, they must set themselves the task of giving special care to the child's teeth. If dental problems are allowed to develop, they will be harder to treat because of the child's other problem.

Children with heart disease, cerebral palsy, mental retardation, and other conditions deserve an extra measure of care. A hemophiliac, for example, who can't take an injection should not have to spend 10 weeks in a hospital for dental care alone before he or she is 8 years old—which can be expected if his or her teeth haven't received careful attention.

When a child is ill, parents tend to become oversolicitous. They will often feed the child constantly, let the child use a bottle as a pacifier, and keep the child on soft foods for a long period of time—all of which will complicate the dental situation.

Think about it. If you've got one serious problem already, you don't need another.

The child with a disability may, when older, need to go more often to the dentist for observation and evaluation. This will bring two benefits:

1. The child learns, through familiarity, to be less anxious and more cooperative at the dentist's office.

2. Frequent checkups reduce the need for extensive treatment, which might involve admitting the child to the hospital for dental treatment under general anesthesia, a costly procedure and a potentially dangerous one. A 2- or 3-year-old is a poor anesthesia risk compared to a 10-year-old. If the choice is made to use anesthesia—and I do sometimes make that choice—you'll want the best possible anesthesiologist because the dentistry is the easy part. It's putting a baby to sleep that's tough.

Review the checklist on page 107. Remember, most dental disease is preventable.

Your baby is now 5 or 6 months old and has a clean, plaque-free mouth; is getting fluoride from drinking water or perhaps is receiving a fluoride supplement; chews vigorously and with evident pleasure when handed a piece of crisp celery or chewy toast; and is beginning to feel little tingly sensations in the ridge of gum in the front of the mouth. Could it be that your child is about to produce a surprise for Mom and Dad and Grandma and Grandpa and all the rest?

Your Child's Teeth From Babyhood Through Adolescence

When Do the First Teeth Appear?

One day your baby will look up at you and smile, and there, most likely in the bottom jaw, gleaming like perfect pearls, will be a couple of brand-new teeth. The first teeth generally come into the mouth when the child is between 6 and 14 months old. They may be the two center front teeth on the bottom, or the two center front on the top—called the incisors. They are small, even, and very white (in fact, so white that when the big, strong, yellowish permanent teeth begin to come in, it will take you a while to get used to the contrast). When all four front incisors are in, the lateral incisors—the very small teeth on either side of the front center teeth—will make their appearance, probably two at a time.

Some children get their teeth early; some children get their teeth late. There's really no medical importance attached to the timing. Every baby's schedule is different, and it may safely vary from the chart on pages 28 and 29. The chart is just to give you an idea of the standard

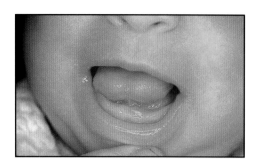

The first tooth generally erupts between 6 months and 1 year of age.

progression, using average ages of eruption. The eruption time of your child's teeth might deviate by as much as 10 to 12 months and still be within the normal range.

There is really no significance to either early or late eruption, except that those children whose teeth erupt later tend to have a slightly higher resistance to dental caries than those whose teeth erupt earlier. In part this is because teeth that stay under gums for a longer time in areas where there is fluoride in the water supply will pick up more fluoride from body tissues before they come out to face the world.

In general, girls' teeth tend to erupt slightly before boys' teeth do. That's no advantage; girls show somewhat more susceptibility than boys to early dental caries, possibly because their teeth have been out longer, exposed to things that can cause decay.

By the time many children are 14 months old, they have four teeth in their mouths. Others of the same age are just beginning to show their first tooth. Keep an eye on what's going on in there. The progression of teething and the number of teeth in your baby's mouth shouldn't be a mystery.

Before your baby is 3 years old, certain things may come to your attention that you'll want to consult a dentist about. Your baby may develop too few teeth. This is sometimes an inherited condition. An examination will reveal if the teeth really are missing or are just late in coming through. Your baby may have too many teeth. If there has been some malformation of the enamel and the teeth look chalky and white with brownish areas, or are soft with yellow spots, special care can be taken to reinforce and save these teeth. Most babies of 18 months have approximately 12 teeth. By the age of 3, the child should have 20 teeth: 10 in the bottom jaw and 10 in the upper jaw. Twenty—count 'em—20. Missing and extra teeth are not uncommon and can easily lead to malocclusions if they are not detected early. Check

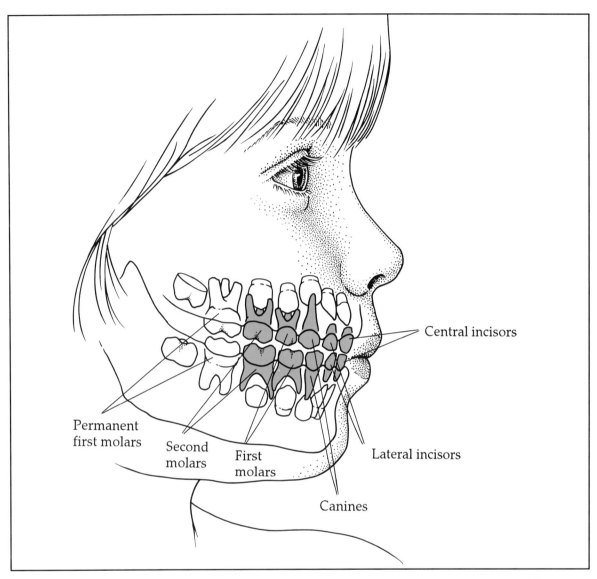

Central incisors

Permanent
first molars

Second
molars

First
molars

Lateral incisors

Canines

This 6-year-old child has all her primary teeth (in blue) and her permanent first molars. The other permanent teeth have not yet erupted.

with your dentist. Teeth can erupt malformed or out of alignment, or not appear at all. Or an early cavity may develop.

The illustration above shows the mouth at 3 years with all 20 primary teeth accounted for. There should be four teeth in between the four pointed canine teeth and then the first and second molars on each side. If there are fewer—or more—after the third birthday, there is reason for concern.

Life Cycle of the Primary (blue) and Permanent Teeth

6 Months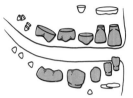

9 Months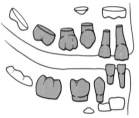

1 Year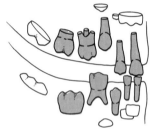

2 Years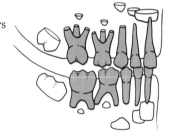

3 Years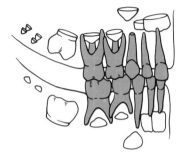

4 Years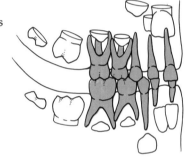

5 Years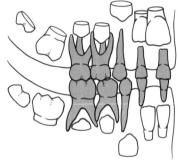

Tooth	When It Arrives (Month)*	When It Leaves (Year)
The upper teeth		
Central incisor	7.5	7
Lateral incisor	9	8
Canine	18	11
First molar	14	9
Second molar	24	11

*Plus or minus 6 months should be considered to be within the normal limit.

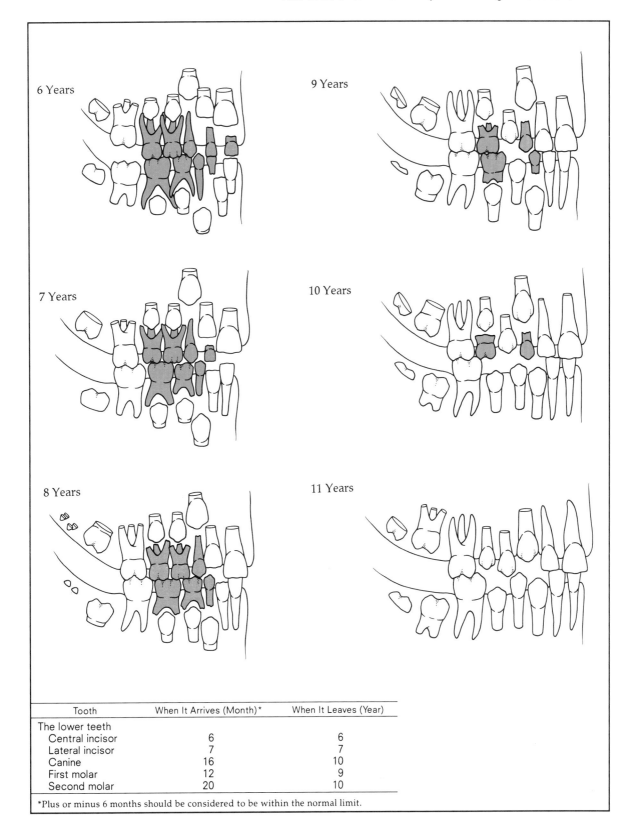

6 Years

7 Years

8 Years

9 Years

10 Years

11 Years

Tooth	When It Arrives (Month)*	When It Leaves (Year)
The lower teeth		
Central incisor	6	6
Lateral incisor	7	7
Canine	16	10
First molar	12	9
Second molar	20	10

*Plus or minus 6 months should be considered to be within the normal limit.

Teething

Although there is wide variation in individual teething patterns, statistics indicate a general progression. The first teeth to come into the mouth are usually the lower central incisors, followed by the top central incisors. The illustration and chart on pages 28 and 29 show the pattern that occurs most frequently. Your baby might vary by several months and there would still be no reason to worry.

Once the central incisors are in, your child will be teething off and on for the next 2 years. Around 9 months, the lateral incisors (the teeth next to the central incisors) arrive. Between 12 and 14 months, the first molars erupt, leaving a gap that the canines will fill at about 18 months. By age 2, the second molars have come in. Then there will be a long waiting period until age 5 or 6, when those very important teeth, the 6-year molars, arrive.

The noted psychoanalyst Erik Erikson has made a guess that the legend of the Garden of Eden, which is told in one version or another by all peoples of the world, goes back to the common preverbal experience when a fussy, cranky, teething baby bites down on his mother's breast, precipitating her decision that it's time to wean the baby and resulting in the child's sense of loss of a paradise.

Teething is only one of the things a baby is going through at the active, adventurous age of 6 months to 1 year. If a 6-month-old has two temper tantrums, throws up on Grandpa's lap, and screams her head off for no apparent reason, the child's parents might be tempted to shrug their shoulders and explain, "She must be teething." It seems as if every time a child whines, drools, cries, or puts things into the mouth, somebody is bound to blame it on teething. And since teeth are erupting off and on from 6 months to 3 years, there would hardly be a time when it couldn't be blamed.

. . . every time a child whines, drools, cries, or puts things into the mouth, somebody is bound to blame it on teething.

Signs That Indicate Teething Is Occurring

If your child is giving some of these signals, take a look in his or her mouth. The first teeth to arrive will be front and center (the four central incisors erupt around the sixth to the tenth month). If the gums here look irritated, red, and puffy, and if you can feel or even see the tip of a tooth coming through, then your baby is teething. If other symptoms show up (fever, nausea, congestion), don't assume that teething is the cause—real sickness is not caused by teething. Check with your pediatrician for other possibilities.

If you don't see any teeth but would like to know where they are, press your thumb firmly on the gum tissue and take it away, quickly; you'll see the shape of the tooth underneath for just a second.

Does Teething Hurt?

There is a great deal of controversy about whether there is any pain associated with teething. There may be none! Teeth don't really "cut" through the gums. The process is one of gradual movement. Teething is a perfectly natural process, running on an individual timetable. In over 30 years of experience as a children's dentist, I have never found it necessary to cut a child's gums to help the primary teeth come through.

There is a great deal of controversy about whether there is any pain associated with teething.

Remedies for Teething Discomfort

If there is some discomfort in teething, different measures seem to relieve it in different babies; you'll find them through experience and observation. I once handed a teething baby a cold, cooked, shelled shrimp, and it worked; but I don't prescribe it, since I don't know whether it was the texture, the temperature, or the novelty of the remedy that worked.

The best thing to do for teething babies is to clean their mouths with a damp gauze pad three or four times a day and give them something to bite on—a teething ring, toast, a chicken drumstick bone stripped of meat. If all else fails, drugstores sell a preparation that can numb your baby's gums.

If your child seems to have a loss of appetite for a while, don't worry. Don't use coercion to get your child to eat. You wouldn't force a pet dog or cat—or an adult, for that matter—to eat if he or she was obviously resisting the idea, would you? Let the child decide.

It is not unusual for healthy children to drool.

Drooling

It is not unusual for healthy children to drool. A young child does not have the muscular control to keep saliva in the mouth. Many things stimulate excessive saliva production: foods, smells, strange tastes, or the irritation that develops around a newly erupted tooth that hasn't been properly cleaned.

Those Important Primary Teeth

Many people still feel that the primary teeth are not important because they are going to fall out anyway. Let's examine that idea a little more carefully.

The 20 primary teeth are designed to function during the childhood years—some of them until the child is 10 or 12 years old—and they have several important jobs to do.

Do you begin to see how important the first teeth are? Instead of thinking of "primary" in its narrow meaning of "first," think of the word as describing a fundamental, basic, important part of an organized whole. Primary teeth are foundation teeth. Early neglect or early loss can result in several problems, and you may as well think about them while you still have a chance to prevent them.

There was a time when dentists thought that all prematurely lost primary teeth had to be replaced, but this isn't so. For example, in the upper front region spaces don't close up. In fact, as children get older and their top jaws get bigger, spaces open up with or without teeth to hold them.

Why the Primary Teeth are Important

- Primary teeth are responsible for maintaining proper spaces for the child's permanent teeth to come into; they serve to guide permanent teeth into position.

- They help in the development of the face and jaws, influencing the growth, height, and shape of the face. How many of us have seen adults whose faces seemed to collapse when they took out their set of dentures? Teeth contribute to one's appearance and sense of self-worth.

- Primary teeth certainly help in the first step of digesting food and, once the baby starts eating more solid fare, in biting and chewing and grinding those foods.

- Healthy, decay-free primary teeth create a healthy environment for the permanent teeth.

But in some areas of the mouth, particularly the back part, the premature loss of a primary tooth will lead to trouble. The adjacent teeth tend to drift into this space; the leaning, crooked teeth will collect more food and be more susceptible to decay. And the tooth that has moved may block a permanent tooth that is waiting to move into that space, or may cause it to erupt at an angle as it tries to find a place for itself. When they erupt into the mouth, teeth don't know where they are going; their resting position is determined by the muscles and other forces that push on them. When the forces are out of balance a malocclusion often develops.

A Look at Primary Teeth

The hard outer coat of the baby's tooth is the enamel, and the part you see is called the crown. The inner, supportive structure, which you cannot see, is the dentin. All of that part of the tooth was formed in the uterus and was in the

Problems With Primary Teeth May Lead to Problems With the Permanent Teeth

- Injuries to the front primary teeth can cause infections and disturbances in the color, shape, and size of the permanent front teeth.

- Of course primary teeth fall out. In fact, the front teeth are kept only 5 or 6 years. But the back primary teeth remain in the mouth for a long time, sometimes until the child is 10 or 12 years old. If these teeth are carrying dental disease, they will pass it right along to the new permanent teeth. If a sound 6-year molar, which is a permanent tooth, erupts into a mouth that is already harboring cavities, it will not take long for the new tooth to be affected, because decay travels fast.

- If a primary tooth becomes infected and abscessed at the root, the infection may damage the underlying permanent tooth.

- If a primary tooth is removed, instead of being filled and saved, expensive braces or space maintainers may be needed to save the space for the unerupted permanent tooth. Whether a space maintainer is needed is a dentist's decision.

- The 6-year molar—the first permanent tooth to appear in the mouth—is going to be the key to the placement of the permanent teeth. It is important, therefore, for the first and second primary molars to be healthy teeth, present and in their normal position, so that this all-important 6-year molar can come into its correct position in the dental arch.

jaw when the baby was born. However, the root, which anchors the tooth and holds it in position, wasn't developed enough to do that job until about the sixth or eighth month after birth. This is all part of nature's timetable.

Color

The color of the first tooth that comes into the mouth is an indication of what the color of all the other teeth is going to be. If the mother was not ill during pregnancy, there is no reason for it not to be a milky white color. If it is some other color, it may indicate a malformation of the enamel, and a dentist should be consulted.

In general, a stained primary tooth probably has the stain not in the tooth but on the outside of the tooth. A stain of this kind often can be removed very easily with a piece of gauze and a little toothpaste.

Mamelons—"Little Bumps"

The first tooth will have small bumps on the biting surface. These are called mamelons. They do not constitute a cutting edge to help the tooth get through the gum, as some people believe. Rather, they are simply the areas where the tooth buds start to develop. A lower incisor will have three or four mamelons on it. In general, these mamelons are worn away as the teeth come into contact with the teeth in the opposing jaw. **Mamelons that have not worn away after a few years are an indication that the teeth are not being used properly. Malocclusion is probably starting to develop. So watch and see if the mamelons start to disappear by the second or third birthday.**

Mamelons that have not worn away after a few years are an indication that the teeth are not being used properly.

Frenum

That little flap of tissue that attaches the center of each lip to the jaw is called the frenum. In some children the flap seems to sit between the permanent incisors, and there may be some space between these two front teeth. A dentist may suggest a *frenectomy*—minor surgery to trim the frenum so that this space can close. In my experience, the need for such surgery is extremely infrequent. This tissue is not necessarily what's keeping the teeth apart.

On rare occasions the frenum is a heavy, tough band—it looks like a rubber band, doubled over—connected on the tongue side. Then it does have to be removed surgically, but it's a simple procedure, with no harmful effects. In the lower jaw, the frenum may be attached right at the neck of the lower incisors. In that position it pulls at the tissue and

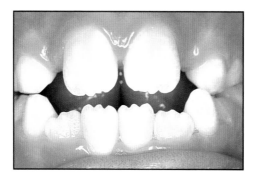

Mamelons, the bumps on the biting edge of these teeth, are normal. As the child gets older, they will wear away.

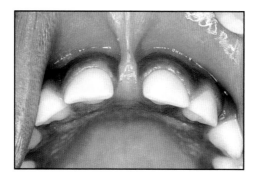

Many people mistakenly believe that it is the frenum (the little flap of tissue that attaches the center of the lip to the jaw) that is keeping the teeth apart. The space between the teeth is normal and will disappear as the child gets older.

is a sufficiently severe problem to require surgical repair. If this is the case, you should have the surgery done when your child is around 9 or 10 years old. Once the child is over age 14 or 15, the periodontal problem is irreversible. A specialist in gum surgery—a *periodontist*—usually does a frenectomy.

Spaces

Does your baby have spaces between the new teeth? It's actually an advantage, because primary teeth with natural separation are less likely to trap food particles and are consequently less susceptible to decay. Nature meant teeth to be self-cleaning: straight, spaced, washed by saliva, and scoured by the coarse, unrefined foods that people ate for centuries. Even if your child's teeth don't seem well spaced when they first come in, you will notice that at about 5 years of age the upper primary teeth begin to spread apart a little. The growing jaw is providing room for the larger permanent teeth, which will eventually take the place of the primary teeth.

Important Milestones in the Growth and Development of Your Child's Teeth

Age  By the first birthday, the bottom and top front teeth have come through the gum and into the mouth, even though the roots are not yet fully formed. The first primary molars are about to appear, and beneath the gums the crowns of the second primary molars are fully formed. Deep in the jaw, the biting surfaces of the first permanent molars are complete, and the first permanent incisors are hardening. The jaw increases in height and width as the cartilage and bone of the jaw grow.

Age By the time the child is 3 years old, all 20 primary teeth are generally present and accounted for, and occlusion (the way the teeth fit together) is being established. Beneath the gums, the crowns of the permanent incisors are almost complete, the permanent canines are about two-thirds complete, and the mineralization of the premolars has just begun. The crowns of the first permanent molars are practically complete; they will slowly rotate forward to face the direction in which they will move through the gums. The roots of all the primary teeth are complete; their pulp chambers are large and the root canals are mature.

Age Your 5-year-old laughs and shows a row of small, white, evenly spaced teeth. Backstage, a lot is going on. Resorption of the roots of the incisors is beginning (resorption is like melting); by the time the incisors loosen and fall out, you'll think these teeth didn't have roots at all, but they did. Now they've been resorbed into the tissue of the gums. That's why the primary teeth fall out when the time comes. The roots of the 5-year-old's permanent incisors are beginning to mineralize, as are the roots of the first permanent molars.

Age First-graders are in for a lot of firsts, among them the first loose tooth and the first smile with a hole in it. By the time the child is 6 years of age, x-rays show that the first permanent molars have rapidly developed and moved up behind the primary molars, their roots more than half formed, and the second permanent molars are moving into position. I find that the first permanent molars are often the first permanent teeth to erupt. Usually parents are not aware that their children already have permanent teeth because they tend to erupt without any discomfort.

The front teeth are lost at about this time. The new, permanent incisors grow through the gum. The permanent canines, lying deeper in the jaws, now have fully formed crowns, and the roots of the other primary teeth continue to be resorbed.

Also at this time, growth in the skull and the upper part of the face is nearly finished, but growth in the lower part of the face is still far from complete. The planes of the face are beginning to take on different dimensions, and your first-grader loses his or her "baby face."

Age The most dramatic changes in dentition have taken place by the time your child is 10. The permanent incisors are fully in. The primary molars are falling out, one by one, and one or more permanent molars are in place. The latecomers—the canines—are undergoing root resorption, and root formation in the permanent canines is taking place. The second permanent molars are ready to come in, and the third molars (the wisdom teeth) are mineralizing. Parents of children who are 9 to 13 years of age are often concerned about the spaces between their children's upper front teeth—so concerned, in fact, that they seek orthodontic help. It may be useful to know that these spaces don't close naturally until the canine teeth erupt and come into occlusion. When they erupt, two out of three youngsters lose the extra space between their top front teeth naturally.

Age When your child is 13, the first and second molars and the canines are in, and the third molars are developing but still under the gum. Except for these last molars, the permanent teeth are complete. The muscles of the mouth and face are growing in order to do the work that will be demanded of them by the adult teeth, and the bones of the face and jaw are reaching adult dimensions and strength. And there are 32 teeth, ready for a lifetime of use.

Cleaning the First Teeth

Children can't clean their own mouths efficiently—any more than they can pick up a pen and write script or cut their food neatly by manipulating their knife and fork. The neural patterns and the muscular coordination that they need for maintaining good hygiene do not develop until they are 8 or 9 years old. So the skills it takes to manipulate the toothbrush and dental floss are just not there. Therefore, you're responsible for keeping your child's mouth clean for a long time. Meanwhile, you're establishing a behavior pattern in both the child and yourself.

Think your own attitude through clearly: This is not something you are doing *to* your child but something you are doing *for* your child. Your child knows the difference. You are not a tyrant, pinning your child to the wall forcibly to brush his or her teeth; you care about your child's body, showing in visible and physical terms that you do, and indicating to your child the importance of learning to value and care for his or her own physical well-being.

Many children are still nursing from a bottle when their teeth begin to come into their mouth. I have already alerted

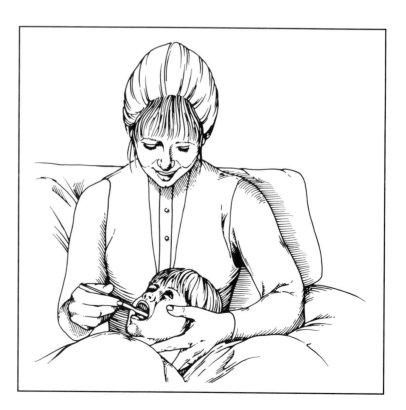

The best position for examining and cleaning a child's teeth.

The Best Way to Examine and Clean Children's Teeth

- Seat yourself on the floor or on a couch or bed, with your child lying in front of you, head in your lap, feet pointing away. This is the best way to clearly see your child's back teeth, both top and bottom. If you try to look in while facing the child directly, the lips and tongue get in the way and you can't see—or brush—effectively.

- Another method of examining a child's mouth is to take a piece of gauze, like the piece you use to wipe the baby's teeth, and put it on the tip of the child's tongue, holding it between your fingers and moving it to the right and left, so that you can get a look.

- Still another way is to use a small pocket flashlight while you hold and move the tongue with a spoon. You'll be surprised at how much you can see.

- If you have difficulty getting the child to open the mouth, slide your forefinger along the inside of the cheek and press down with the ball of your finger behind the last tooth on the bottom.

- It's a simple matter, and it can be fun, to check the number of teeth and their color, see if surfaces are clean, and help your child with brushing. I'm always amazed at the number of parents who bring their children to my office who have never themselves looked at their children's teeth.

you to the dangers of pacifying children with a nursing bottle—that is, letting them nurse for long periods or take a bottle of juice or milk into their bed at night. There is really no need to feed children constantly. Aren't they getting an adequate diet at mealtime?

Once the teeth start to erupt into the mouth, as early as 4 months of age, they should be cleaned twice a day—after breakfast and before bedtime—exactly as you've been cleaning the gum pads.

Position your child as shown on page 38 and wipe both surfaces—front and back—of the teeth and gum pads. As other teeth erupt into the mouth, clean gum pads will keep the area clean and free of food particles and will cut down on the number of bacteria in the mouth.

Use a tiny dab of fluoride toothpaste on a gauze pad held between your fingers. Or try some of the new oral hygiene products for infants, including wipes, toothbrushes, and toothpastes designed specifically for young children.

At some point—after the incisors are in—you'll want to graduate to a small toothbrush with a straight, small head and even, soft bristles. You will still have to do most of the brushing for some time.

When Should Children Be Able to Brush Their Own Teeth?

Few children before the age of 5 can do an adequate job of cleaning their mouths.

My experience has always been that parents want their children to be independent and take care of their own teeth. Instinctively—more important, culturally—parents don't want to feel responsible for cleaning their children's teeth. When I counsel parents I suggest to them, "Look at it this way— you're helping your child to reach a point where he or she can manage alone."

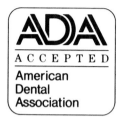

Look for this statement of acceptance by the ADA when shopping for toothpaste.

As children approach their second birthday, they can be introduced to using a toothbrush themselves. However, this is just to get them into the habit of holding the toothbrush and brushing—a good habit to develop. Good dental habits established with the primary teeth will usually be carried over into the care of the permanent teeth. But for now, it is still the parents' job and responsibility to keep their child's mouth clean.

Use a little fluoride toothpaste on a child's toothbrush, and try to teach the child not to swallow toothpaste. The most important function of a good modern toothpaste is to carry topical fluoride. The more often fluoride comes in contact with the tooth, the stronger that tooth is going to be. This is important protection that will supplement the fluoride in drinking water.

You can tell if a commercial toothpaste containing fluoride is reputable by looking on the box for a statement of acceptance by the Council on Dental Therapeutics of the American Dental Association (ADA).

Mouthwashes versus Fluoride Mouthrinses

Traditional commercial mouthwashes are of limited value to your child's dental health. In general, they do little more than freshen the mouth temporarily. For ordinary rinsing, plain water is a terrific mouthwash.

Fluoride mouthrinses, on the other hand, are a relatively recent development that provide another valuable source of topical fluoride. They can be particularly beneficial for children who are highly susceptible to cavities or who are wearing orthodontic braces. (Braces make toothbrushing more challenging for even the most skilled children, and that puts them at increased risk for cavities.)

Fluoride mouthrinses come in different forms: some are meant to be swallowed, most are meant to be swished around and spat out. Be sure you know which kind you are buying and what your child is doing with it.

Should children under age 5 routinely use a fluoride mouthrinse? There is some disagreement among professionals on this point. Up until about age 6, most children lack sufficient control to swish and spit; they are more likely to swallow the stuff. For that reason, I recommend that you ask your own dentist for advice on whether your child should use fluoride mouthrinse.

If you then decide to add fluoride mouthrinse to your child's daily routine, have your child use it right after brushing.

Bad Breath

There is no dental reason for a child with a daily teeth-cleaning routine to have bad breath (halitosis). The problem is more likely to originate in the stomach or small intestine than in a clean mouth. In an adult, bad breath may be an indication of plaque accumulation, but when a child has bad breath, you should suspect that some other problem is responsible. It's not coming from the teeth. A child with bad breath either had garlic for dinner the evening before or is suffering from some gastric or other medical problem, which should be investigated carefully.

. . . when a child has bad breath, you should suspect that some other problem is responsible. It's not coming from the teeth.

Sealants: Long-Lasting Dental "Insurance"

Pit and fissure sealants are a special liquid plastic that dentists use to literally coat the most cavity-prone tooth surfaces and shield them from decay. Studies have shown that four out of five cavities form on the chewing surfaces of the back teeth—precisely where long-lasting sealant protection can be applied.

Sealants are available in clear or tinted versions (more easily visible), and have been proven over two decades to dramatically reduce cavities in the most vulnerable tooth surfaces. **I believe it's a good idea to buy your youngster some added security: have your dentist apply sealant to all your child's molar teeth—primary and permanent—as soon as possible after they erupt.**

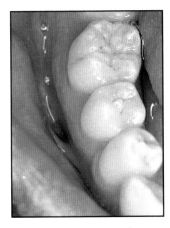

Before sealant is applied.

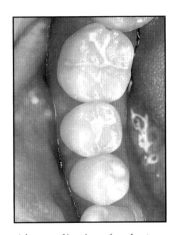

After application of sealant.

Tooth Position and Bad Habits

Will Your Child's Teeth Erupt in an Ideal Alignment?

We talk about the primary teeth "erupting" into the mouth, but that is really a rather violent word for the process. Eruption is more of a gliding, sliding movement, with the teeth advancing slowly through the gums, and the gums thinning and parting to allow the advance. There is no such thing as "eruptive force." The "force" that brings a tooth into the mouth is a development of the bone surrounding each individual tooth bud.

If you are watching your child's mouth so that you are aware of the arrival of the primary teeth, and if you're familiar with the chart on pages 28 and 29, showing the pattern of eruption, then you are probably hoping that your child's teeth are going to line up in an ideal arrangement in the dental arch. However, the position that the tooth assumes in the dental arch is determined by the forces that act on the tooth once it has erupted through the gums. These forces include:

- Tongue movements that push
- Lip movements that hold in
- Movements of cheek muscles
- Pressure that occurs when the tooth meets an opposing tooth in the other jaw
- Atmospheric pressure that affects the tooth every time the child swallows or closes the mouth

It is possible by examining the position of the teeth in the primary dentition to get a fair idea of the various forces that are going to act on the permanent teeth when they start to erupt into the mouth, about the time the child is 6 or 7 years old. Forces that push the primary teeth toward faulty closure will probably have to be dealt with in the arrangement of the permanent teeth.

If, when the jaw is closed, the child has a steep overbite (the upper teeth come forward and cover the lower line of teeth), or the midlines are not parallel (the gap between the two front top teeth does not line up with the gap between the two front bottom teeth), there may be a pernicious habit that is exerting pressure in your child's mouth. Let's describe some of these habits, and then you can check your family out.

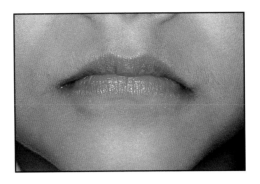

This is what the lips look like when a child has a lip-biting habit.

Bad Habits—How to Recognize Them and What to Do About Them

Many malocclusions are caused by an imbalance in the pressures of the muscle systems that are guiding the teeth into position or holding them in position where they belong. It is possible, when we're made aware of them, to detect the presence of bad habits that create this imbalance before they have an opportunity to affect the developing teeth and before the habits result in a fixed musculature pattern that the child may continue to repeat for the rest of his or her life.

Lip Biting

One of the earliest and most common of all habits causing malocclusion is lip biting. There is no reason for a well child to have chapped lips, even during the winter. If your child has chapped lips—especially a chapped lower lip—check for lip biting.

Most parents are unaware that their child is engaging in such a habit. But inspection of a child's lips even at 2 years of age will show a tendency toward lip biting if it exists: look to see if the red portion of the lower lip is larger than the upper lip. In school, a child sitting and biting his or her lip looks rather thoughtful and studious. We may not recognize this as a pernicious habit at first. In little girls it is often attractive and thought of as a "pouty" look. However, close examination of the vermilion border (the lip line) of the lower lip will show it to be diffuse, with no sharp demarcation between the pink and the red.

I'd almost rather see children suck their thumbs than bite their lower lips. There's a lot of social pressure on thumb suckers, from family and peers, that keeps them from

One of the earliest and most common of all habits causing malocclusion is lip biting.

exercising the habit all the time, while lip biters look preoccupied and no one thinks to discourage the habit.

As the lip gets dry from having its natural oils removed by the tongue, it tends to itch. Children have a tendency to pull it up inside their mouth and scratch it with their upper teeth and then wet it again. As they wet it they take the oils out of the skin, which dries up and becomes chapped and irritated. They then tend to scratch the lip again with their upper teeth, wet their lip with their tongue, and allow it to dry out. They keep repeating these actions.

An emollient (such as a lip balm, petroleum jelly, or cold cream) placed on the part of the lip the child bites can be used to help a child break a lip-biting habit. This is soothing, and there won't be quite so much urge to scratch the lip because it won't feel dry and itchy. It takes many months to break a habit once it is formed, so it's best to start working on it as soon as the habit is detected. Be aware of the possibility of such habits being formed by your child very early, especially before the third year.

Tongue Thrusting

Tongue thrusting is one of the most difficult muscular habits with which the dentist has to deal. If it could be prevented, many difficult orthodontic cases would be self-correcting.

Observe your child quietly and unobtrusively. If your child has a tongue-thrust habit, each time he or she swallows the tongue will be pushed forward between the upper and lower teeth when they are in occlusion. Another clue is a wrinkling between the child's lower lip and chin when swallowing.

A child who is a tongue thruster will have to learn to swallow correctly. Have your child practice by eating or drinking while sitting in front of a mirror and watching to see that he or she doesn't "wrinkle up" with each swallow.

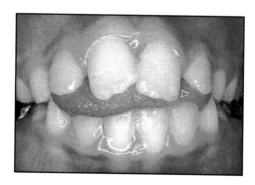

This type of "open bite" occurs in children with a tongue thrusting habit.

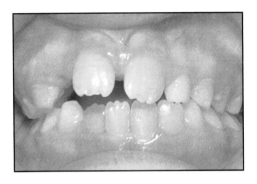

Teeth of a child with a fingernail-biting habit. Notice how the lower teeth are turned.

Fingernail Biting

Many children start to bite on their fingernails when they are as young as 2 years. Parents who find that they never have to cut their child's fingernails may be in the best position to diagnose the habit. Fingernail biting usually causes the rotations that we see in the teeth in the anterior section of the mouth. It may also contribute to a slight wearing away of the biting surfaces, and of course it introduces germs and dirt into the mouth.

As with any habit, aroused self-awareness, helpful reminders—and in this case perhaps, social disapproval from peers—contribute to its breaking.

Cheek Biting

First, look inside your child's mouth for a swollen flap of skin. Cheek biting is one of the most difficult habits for parents to detect. Because it occurs only when the teeth are together and the mouth is closed, you'll have to watch for outside signs of interior movement in order to detect the presence of the habit. Point out to the child what he or she is doing, and help the child to watch for its recurrence.

Tooth Grinding

Tooth grinding (the dental term is *bruxism*) probably starts even before the first tooth comes into the mouth. There is a tendency in some children to gnash their upper and lower jaws together while sleeping and sometimes while at rest during the day. It is an expression of a muscular habit that serves as a tension-releasing device. As their teeth start coming into the mouth, children who are bruxists can

Parents who find that they never have to cut their child's fingernails may be in the best position to diagnose the [fingernail biting] habit.

make a considerable amount of noise by grinding their teeth when in bed.

Bruxism alone does not cause malocclusion, but it can tend to delay the loss of the primary teeth. The permanent teeth have a much more difficult time coming into the mouth when bruxism is practiced. The time of their eruption may be delayed, the sequence of eruption is often disturbed, and malocclusion may result from these interferences.

Children who are confirmed bruxists will probably do little to their primary teeth with all that grinding, except keep them extremely clean and prevent cavities, since they wear the teeth away faster than they can decay. But bruxists must be watched extremely carefully when it comes time for them to lose their primary teeth. Tell your dentist if your child is a tooth grinder, and be prepared to have some primary teeth removed if they do not fall out at the correct time. To my knowledge, there's no known way of breaking the habit of bruxism. (Appliances worn at night ["bite guards"] do little more than cut down on the noise; they are not well-accepted and are generally lost by the child — "accidentally, on purpose.") Sometimes, when the tooth-grinding habit persists until children have their permanent teeth, it's associated with periodontal disease and jaw problems.

Bad Habit "Checkup"

Use these tips as a guide for detecting the most common bad habits that can affect your child's dental health.

Lip biting: Chapped lips; lower lip larger than upper lip

Tongue Thrusting: Muscles over chin wrinkling when child swallows

Nail biting: No need to cut nails

Cheek biting: Swollen flap of tissue inside cheek

Finger biting: Callus on finger

Thumb sucking: A clean thumb

Keeping a Mouthful of Things

Objects such as blanket corners, shoelaces, shirt sleeves, toys, and so forth are used by children as substitutes for their thumbs and as pacifiers for biting and chewing. Used for short periods of time, none of these is dangerous. (Think of the substitutes we adults use: cigarettes, cigars, gum, pencils, pipes.) However, when children keep one of these in their mouths for many hours a day, malocclusion generally results. It's true that all children should be allowed to bite and chew and suck and to enjoy these oral activities, but they should be discouraged from doing any of these things constantly, hour after hour, day after day.

About Pacifiers

In general, I find pacifiers an important outlet and I recommend that parents not do anything about them. The energy expended by a child on a pacifier often finds its expression, when it is displaced, in other more objectionable types of behavior—for example, temper tantrums or bedwetting.

Most children give up the pacifier habit on their own, without parental intervention, by age 3 or 4. Until then, I believe Linus should be permitted to have his security blanket; I don't believe in taking it away from him.

But if children cling to the habit into their fourth or fifth year, you may need to intervene. To stop this or any other habit, you must first bring it to a conscious level. Gently but consistently remind the child that he or she is engaging in the habit each time it occurs. Don't belittle and don't make a big deal of it. Don't imply, for instance, that "bad children suck their thumbs, good children do not." No rewards. Just stay loose and remember that eventually most children get the idea.

I do not use mechanical means to prevent children from engaging in such habits as thumb sucking. I will sometimes make them an appliance that acts as a reminder not to suck the thumb. It doesn't punish or even prevent; the thumb just doesn't feel the way it used to. Children generally give up the habit when they don't get the old biofeedback.

A Final Word on Eradicating Bad Habits

Lip sucking, tongue thrusting, nail biting, cheek biting— these are habits that, like thumb and finger sucking for infants and toddlers, may serve emotional needs. Try to evaluate the habit before you begin a campaign to get rid of

> *To stop any habit, you must first bring it to a conscious level.*

My Best Suggestions for Breaking Bad Habits

Step 1: Understand, first, that a habit is an unconscious muscular pattern. It must be brought to conscious attention before it can be dealt with. If your child sucks his thumb, tell him so: "Billy, you're sucking your thumb." Don't be negative—he has no control over the habit because he doesn't know he's sucking. It may take 3 or 4 months before Billy knows that he's putting his thumb in his mouth.

Step 2: After Billy understands that he has a habit, and agrees that it would be better not to stick his thumb in his mouth, you may suggest aids that will remind him—anything from an appliance made by a dentist to a piece of tape placed on the thumb as a reminder, or a sock on the hand when he goes to sleep. However, if you use any of these aids before Billy is aware of the habit or agrees that he really wants to drop it, you are going to do more harm than good.

Habits such as tongue thrusting and lip biting take a long time to break— perhaps as long as 2 or 3 years. But the effort is well worth it. It takes no longer than the orthodontics that may be ahead if the habit is not left behind by the maturing child.

it. Is it a mannerism or positional habit that the child, with encouragement and reminding, is ready to give up? Is it a habit hanging on from early childhood, which new status as a "big kid" will help lay to rest? Or is it a compulsive habit connected with some deep emotional need on the child's part? You may have to decide to let the underlying need express itself in a "bad" habit—even though orthodontic treatment will later be needed to correct the results—on the grounds that crooked teeth are easier to straighten than a warped personality.

Speech and Teeth

For many years dentists and speech pathologists felt that the teeth were essential in helping children speak and pronounce word sounds. Children who lisped or had trouble with their dental sounds—d's, t's—were thought to be having trouble with their teeth. Parents have come to my office to ask if teeth are related to some speech problem their child is having.

To my knowledge, there does not seem to be such a relationship. If a youngster at the age of 4 or 5 loses the four primary incisors because of a fall, or has to have them extracted for some reason, his or her speech pattern does indeed change—for 2 or 3 weeks. After that, the child sounds exactly as before.

The same thing happens when a child wears an appliance. If a dentist makes an appliance for a child to discourage a thumb-sucking habit or to move anterior teeth back, the child's speech pattern alters for a couple of days, then returns to normal as the child's mouth adjusts.

I believe most speech problems are not tooth-related. I think it's what the child hears, in addition to a combination of muscular movements. I have seen children recommended for orthodontics when speech pathologists became frustrated and hoped that changing the position of the tongue or tooth or lip was going to solve the problem. I wish dentists could help in this area, but the answer is not in our hands.

. . . most speech problems are not tooth-related.

Cleaning Techniques as Your Child Grows Older

(See also Chapter 4)

Toothbrushes

As the molars start to come into the mouth, cleaning the little grooves and crevices on the surfaces of the molar teeth is too difficult a job for a little square of gauze to do. So, if your child hasn't graduated to a toothbrush yet, now is the time. It really doesn't matter whether you use a nylon- or natural-bristle toothbrush with a child. The objective is getting the food particles and plaque off the teeth. A brush with a small head, a straight handle, and a flat soft-bristle brushing surface is fine. It's a good idea to have two brushes, so that one is always dry and ready for use.

If you have been spending time cleaning your child's mouth and watching the teeth come in, you will know when they are dirty. It is still necessary, until children are around 5, for you to help them to brush their teeth twice a day—after breakfast and before bedtime. Parents could alternate the duty, with one taking the responsibility in the morning and the other in the evening, as it fits their schedules.

It is still necessary, until children are around age 5, for you to help them to brush their teeth twice a day . . .

It's particularly hard for a young child to clean the back teeth.

Another good use of the toothbrush is for brushing the top surface of the tongue. The top of the tongue is covered with the same tissue as that which covers the teeth and gum pads—literally, the skin of your teeth. Brushing the tongue once in a while is a great help in reducing the number of oral bacteria and plaque-forming organisms.

While it's important to encourage your child to use a toothbrush alone, remember that it is your responsibility to keep the child's teeth clean. It's particularly hard for a young child to clean the back teeth. The best way to reach these teeth is to cradle the child's head in the crook of your arm while making a back-and-forth brushing stroke on the biting surfaces of the child's teeth, followed by a whisking up-and-down stroke on the tongue and on the cheek sides. Look at the illustration on page 38, showing how to examine your child's teeth. This position is good for toothbrushing, too.

A soft-scrub technique that you and your child can master easily is described step-by-step in Chapter 4.

An electric toothbrush, when used correctly, is more efficient in cleaning the teeth than a standard toothbrush. But children who are not accustomed to having a standard toothbrush used in their mouth are not likely to tolerate the use of an electric toothbrush.

Many parents purchase electric toothbrushes for their children in the hope that they will use them, but in a few days the novelty wears off. If children do not have the habit of brushing their teeth routinely with a regular brush, they are not going to be able to make the transition to the electric model, and parents who hope their children will are only deluding themselves.

Mouthwashes and Mouthrinses

No evidence exists that the routine use of a mouthwash will cut down on the number of colds children get or that it will be at all beneficial in helping children recover from a cold that they may have at the time. Using a mouthwash does not—repeat, does not—remove food particles from between the teeth, nor does it eliminate bad breath. It only masks it, just as a flavored toothpaste does, for short periods of time.

However, don't confuse an adult mouthwash with a child's fluoride mouthrinse; they are different, and the difference is important. Fluoride mouthrinses bring fluoride in contact with the tooth. If your child uses one, it should be used at the end of the cleaning routine.

Toothpastes

A toothpaste acts primarily as a carrier for detergent and for fluoride. Many people go merrily through life without ever using one. This is certainly permissible. Salt and water or baking soda and water are also excellent for cleaning the teeth. Many individuals choose to brush their teeth with water and nothing else. The object, after all, is to remove debris from the teeth.

Young children, especially around age 2, should be watched carefully to ensure that they do not swallow fluoride toothpaste.

If you want your child to use a toothpaste, you have many from which to choose. Manufacturers are offering more options, many aimed specifically at enticing your child to brush. So, there are toothpastes with colors, stripes, or sparkles, nonfoaming toothpastes, and toothpastes flavored to appeal to kids. There are also fluoride and no-fluoride formulas.

As a rule, I recommend using an ADA-approved fluoride toothpaste, but please consult your child's dentist for advice. Before making a recommendation, the dentist will take into consideration many factors, such as whether your child drinks fluoridated water, juice, and soft drinks, and whether he or she tends to swallow toothpaste.

Water-Irrigating Devices

Water-irrigating devices (Water Pik® is one brand) are a lot of fun. Functionally, they are excellent tools for wetting the bathroom floor, mirror, and pajamas. They are useful, too, for those who have braces, bridges, and other equipment in their mouths.

Because you find that a water jet feels good, you can't understand why everybody shouldn't use one. But you are a grown-up, dealing perhaps with gum problems as well as bridges and caps. Children don't get the same physical sensation because they don't have the same situation.

Water jets do little to remove dental plaque from teeth. Primary teeth and young permanent teeth generally have spaces between them and do not collect food, so the use of a water-irrigating device to remove particles of food is of little value in children. Teenagers, however, may find these devices helpful in cleaning their erupting wisdom teeth (see page 65).

Dental Floss

It is difficult, if not impossible, to reach the plaque between all teeth at all times with the aid of a toothbrush. The only way to clean between the teeth adequately is by rubbing or buffing those areas with a piece of dental floss. By shining the neighboring surfaces of each tooth with dental floss, you'll be able to remove the plaque, bacteria, and food that harbor there and prevent the caries that forms between these teeth. It's a good idea to floss at least once a day.

In a child, there are four spots that need regular flossing. They are between the last two molars on each side of each jaw. Try to make flossing these four sites part of the evening cleaning routine. Again, you'll have to do it until your child can handle it alone. (See Chapter 4 for proper flossing technique.)

In a child, there are four spots that need regular flossing.

Green, Black, Orange Stains

Inside, outside: green, black, orange. At different intervals in the developing dentition, a child's teeth may develop strange colors.

Tetracycline Stain

In the late 1950s and early 1960s, the drug tetracycline was a popular antibiotic for children and adults. Physicians and pediatricians used it to treat infections, especially those accompanied by fevers. The problem: tetracycline is a dye that will stain any tissue that is mineralizing (forming) at the time of its use. If a pregnant woman takes it, it will stain the teeth that are forming in the baby in utero. When the child's primary teeth come in, they often look yellow or orange.

Some young children who were given the drug between birth and 5 years had their developing permanent teeth stained. Today their teeth are dark gray to yellow to orange.

What can be done about it?

Now that we know what the effects are, we don't give children and pregnant women this drug. Other antibiotics are available. Most pediatricians know this, but it doesn't hurt for parents to ask what drug is being given to their child. You may have a pediatrician who got his or her training in the 1950s and thinks of tetracycline as a reliable drug that has worked in the past.

A tooth with a green, yellow, or orange cast is considered a tetracycline-stained tooth. To identify such teeth, look at a history of medications the child has been given, and test the teeth by shining an ultraviolet light on them. They will give off a greenish-orange glow if the stain was caused by tetracycline.

The old treatment—bleaching the teeth over a period of months with a peroxide solution and strong light—has proved ineffective. It doesn't last. Today, some dentists are combining bleaching with enamel microabrasion and achieving more promising results.

For many years now, dentists have been using a tooth-colored, thin plastic veneer that can be attached over stained, fractured, or crooked teeth to correct their appearance. The procedure is painless, fast, and gives extremely good results. (See photographs on pages 60 and 61.)

Green Stain

Green teeth usually occur in the upper jaw in the front of the mouth at the gum line. This condition is caused by plants called algae—the same algae you find in your fish tank. They grow only where there is light, that is, in the front of the mouth, on the top front teeth, and they grow at the gum line, where the climate is moist and they can obtain food. Parents can remove the green stain at home by taking a piece of gauze, placing a little toothpaste or baking soda on it, and scrubbing away just where the tooth meets the gum line. The green color doesn't mean the teeth are impaired, but it does make the teeth look odd.

Black Stain

Black stain (sometimes called *pellicle*) develops in a number of children. You'll notice it, if it exists, as dark, black lines running front and back along the gum line of most of the teeth. It forms when the surface of the tooth becomes stained by some of the salts that occur naturally in the saliva. It is difficult to remove by mechanical means, that

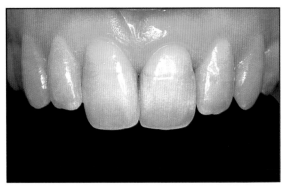 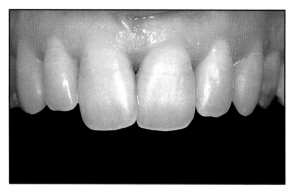

These before-and-after photographs illustrate successful bleaching treatment of previously stained teeth.

is, with a toothbrush or a piece gauze and toothpaste. It can be removed in a dentist's office with a rotating rubber polishing cup. However, it re-forms rather quickly. Pellicle tends to disappear as the permanent teeth come into the mouth and the child reaches 9 or 10 years of age. In some ways you are lucky if your child has this stain, for children who have pellicle tend to develop few dental cavities. Exactly what the relationship is between black stain and dental cavities, nobody yet knows.

White teeth are not necessarily healthy teeth.

Orange Stain

Orange stain is usually found at the gum line in upper and lower teeth. It is caused by color-producing (*chromogenic*) bacteria. Why some children have these orange-colored bacteria and some don't have them is not known. It is thought that the golden- or orange-colored bacteria tend to grow in children who drink a lot of milk. This stain, too, can be removed at home with a gauze pad and a little bit of toothpaste rubbed vigorously at the gum line. Children with chromogenic bacteria are often highly susceptible to dental caries. If children have a colony of "orange bugs" growing on their front teeth, it usually means that some-body is falling down on the job of helping them clean their teeth.

White teeth are not necessarily healthy teeth. Your child's adult teeth may come through looking much yellow-er than the milky white primary teeth, or they may have an ivory cast. This is natural, in spite of the movie-star flash of white we are conditioned to admire. In fact, whiteness may indicate a soft, porous enamel.

The Most Important Teeth: The 6-Year Molars

At about the age of 6, your child's first permanent tooth arrives in the mouth: the 6-year molar. Because it does not replace a lost baby tooth but comes in behind the second primary molar, some parents do not realize that it's a permanent tooth. But you'll know because you've been checking and counting and familiarizing yourself with your child's first set of teeth.

If there has been no premature loss of primary teeth, the 6-year molars will come into the mouth in proper place. (One of the jobs primary teeth perform is stabilizing the position of permanent teeth.) These 6-year molars are probably the most important teeth in the mouth. If they are in their proper place, they act as foundations for the dental arch and keep all the other teeth in their proper positions. A dentist can often take a look at the way the 6-year molars fit in the arch and predict whether the bite (occlusion) is going to be normal.

When the four new permanent 6-year molars are in place, each in its corner of the jaws, they hold the jaws in position in relation to each other while the primary teeth are being shed—another example of nature's timing. The teeth hold this height while the primary teeth in front are being lost, and they also serve as natural space maintainers for the permanent second (12-year) molars that will come in behind them.

If any teeth in the mouth are to be guarded and protected, it is these 6-year molars. If a cavity forms, it should be repaired promptly. And I can hardly imagine a situation in which a 6-year molar should be extracted. Such a step can lead to complex and expensive orthodontic corrections or permanent problems in the position and fit of the teeth. Cherish that tooth! Unfortunately, its biting surface is the most likely place for a cavity to develop. Your dentist should always apply a protective layer of plastic sealant on the biting surface of the 6-year molar as added insurance against cavities (See Chapter 4).

I can hardly imagine a situation in which a 6-year molar should be extracted . . . Unfortunately, its biting surface is the most likely place for a cavity to develop.

What To Do About a Loose Primary Tooth: Just Pull It Out!

When primary teeth become loose, they will often hang on in the front or back of the mouth for weeks at a time,

"When a child loses a primary tooth, the Tooth Fairy comes at night and takes the tooth from under the pillow, leaving a coin in its place."

True. This has happened in experiment after experiment, in generations of families. Dentists are at a loss to explain this scientifically, but they reassure patients that anything that makes losing primary teeth a little more fun is dentally okay.

becoming painful to chew on and irritating to the gums. Parents are at a loss to know what to do.

My advice is to take the tooth between two fingers, give it a sharp tug, and take it out. There's probably little pain in this quick yank—no more than in pulling out a single hair—a short sensation, soon gone. The pain was from the loose tooth's being pushed against soft tissue. If any bleeding occurs afterward, you can control it with pressure by holding a little piece of cotton or gauze on the gum for a few minutes.

Too often, parents come into my office with a child who has had a loose primary tooth for a week or two; the gum is sore and inflamed. But there's no need to wait that long. Be brave. Go ahead and pull it. If it's not loose enough, it won't come out. If you really can't bear to do the job with a stubborn tooth, take the child to the dentist, who will flow a few drops of an anesthetic solution directly next to the tooth and then lift it out painlessly.

If a loose primary tooth inadvertently gets swallowed, don't worry. The enamel will not be digested. And the tooth will pass right through the digestive tract like a seed or cherry pit. Children swallow things like that all the time.

Injuries and Traumas

I suppose one of the most upsetting things—to parent and child—is an accident in which a child's tooth is fractured, displaced, or knocked out. It's painful for the child and an emergency situation for the parent.

The majority of these injuries result from simple accidents—minor falls, sports mishaps, childish pranks. As you may guess, they most often involve the front teeth, so in addition to pain and discomfort, there's the problem of appearance.

Although many accidents befall the toddler, statistics show that children aged 9 and 10 are the most susceptible to damage, and boys are about twice as likely as girls to have such an accident.

Always use seat belts or child-safety seats in your automobile to avoid accidental injury to the face, head, and teeth. And have your child wear a mouth guard when he or she participates in contact sports.

Mouth Guards

If your child participates in sports, a properly fitted mouth guard is essential. More important than a new baseball glove, the latest high-tech roller skates, or the trendiest athletic footwear, mouth guards are top-priority sporting equipment. They protect not only the teeth, but also the lips, cheeks, and tongue. They may even provide protection from such head-and-neck injuries as concussions and jaw fractures.

But a mouth guard only protects when it's worn! Your child should wear a mouth guard for any activity that might involve possible falls, head contact, or flying objects. That includes football, baseball, basketball, soccer, hockey, skateboarding, and gymnastics.

If your child balks at wearing protective mouth gear, point out that the top pro and amateur athletes swear by them. In fact, many professional and school coaches insist that their players wear mouth guards or they don't play, period.

Today's mouth guard options range from (the less desirable) off-the-rack, "boil-to-fit" styles to custom-made appliances available from your dentist. You can buy mouth guards in a variety of colors and even have them personalized with the child's name. And a properly fitted device won't interfere with speaking—you can even sing while wearing one, if the mood strikes.

A custom-fitted mouth guard is a bit more expensive but is well worth it. Because the device is tailor-made to fit your child's mouth, it's far more comfortable to wear. That means your child is more likely to wear it, which makes it far more effective protection than an appliance that sits in the gym locker gathering dust.

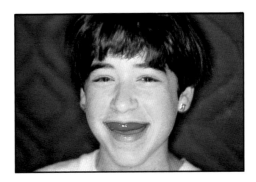

Your child should wear a mouth guard when participating in any contact sports.

Hidden Damage

Any injury that damages a primary tooth has the potential to damage the developing permanent teeth, especially if the injury occurs before age 3. That's why it's important to report *any* such injury promptly to your child's dentist.

The permanent top central incisors begin mineralization at birth and take about 3 years to completely form. If during this critical time the root of a primary tooth is pushed into the developing crown of a permanent tooth, a defect can develop in the permanent tooth.

Don't be surprised, then, if a pediatric dentist recommends *removing* a primary tooth following an injury to an infant's tooth. If removal may help prevent infection or injury to the developing permanent tooth, the dentist will likely advise this treatment—even if it makes the parents feel guilty and unhappy. Remember, loss of a top front tooth in a child under 3 generally does not affect speech, growth patterns, or psychologic development. Children are not tooth conscious until 5 or 6 years of age. And by that time, all their friends are losing their front teeth anyhow.

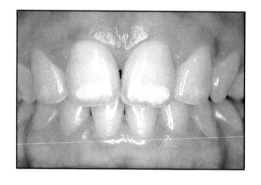

The white spot defects on this adolescent's permanent teeth were caused by an injury to the primary teeth at 18 months of age.

What to Do in Case of an Injury

Sometimes a fall or other injury will knock a tooth out completely. The best thing to do is to wipe the tooth free of dirt (rinse under cold water if necessary) and stick it firmly back in the socket—as far as it will go. Some parents can't bring themselves to do this, but if the tooth isn't back in the mouth within, at most, 20 minutes, the chance of success-ful reimplantation diminishes rapidly. Because play-grounds, schoolyards, and swimming pools rarely provide on-site emergency dental care, you might be called on to perform such first aid.

The next best way to transport a tooth that has been knocked out of a child's mouth is to have the child hold the tooth in the mouth under the tongue until the dentist places it back in its correct position. The saliva in the mouth provides the best emergency environment.

Even if the tooth isn't back in place within 20 minutes, all is not lost. Get the tooth (which should be kept damp) and child to a dentist or to a hospital or medical center emer-gency room with a dentist on duty. Depending on the condition of the tooth and child, the dentist may be able to replace the tooth in the mouth. Sometimes a reimplanted tooth will give several more years of service. If a reim-planted primary tooth lasts 1 to 3 years, that's all the time you need before the underlying permanent tooth is ready to take its place. If the reimplanted tooth is a permanent one, it may last a few years before beginning to die. Then the root will resorb and the tooth will loosen and fall out. No one has figured out how to arrest the process, although many—including me—are trying different implantation techniques.

In an accident that results in a fractured or chipped tooth in which the tooth stays in the mouth, you should wipe the tooth with warm water, keep it clean, and as soon as possible get your child to a dentist, who can place a covering over the exposed tooth structure and thus give the tooth time to heal.

With fractured permanent teeth, there have been amaz-ing advances in repair. In the past, a dentist would cut the tooth down and put a cap on it. Today, there are tooth-colored materials that can be bonded directly to the tooth, without the use of anesthesia and without any cutting of the tooth structure. Liquid quartz is one of these materials and is the same material used to fix teeth with stains caused by tetracycline. Many young people who have chips and cracks in their front teeth, or spaces between them, are being treated with this material. I see many teenagers in my practice who have spent 6 or 7 years feeling self-conscious about a damaged tooth, and after just one office visit they leave with a restoration that is indistinguishable from a natural, whole tooth.

I see many teenagers . . . who have spent 6 or 7 years feeling self-conscious about a damaged tooth, and after one office visit they leave with a restoration that is indistinguishable from a natural, whole tooth.

Cosmetic Dentistry for Children and Adolescents

These before-and-after photographs show how a tooth-colored plastic material enables dentists to restore and reshape front teeth without cutting the tooth to make room for a filling material or a cap. The material is bonded directly to the tooth.

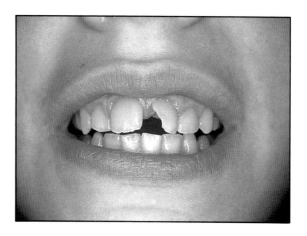

While playing hockey, this 12-year-old boy fractured his upper left central incisor. Fortunately, the nerves of the tooth were not exposed, and his dentist was able to bond a tooth-colored plastic restorative material directly to the tooth. It is almost impossible to distinguish the repaired tooth from the originals.

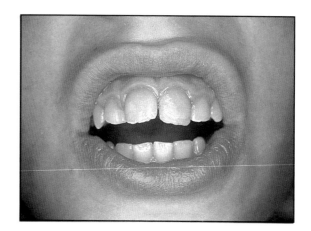

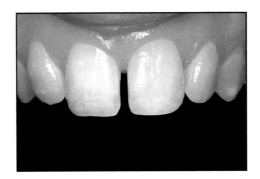

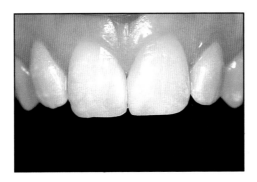

This 14-year-old girl was unhappy with the large space between her upper two front teeth. Her dentist closed the gap by applying a bit of restorative material to each tooth. She is now pleased with her smile.

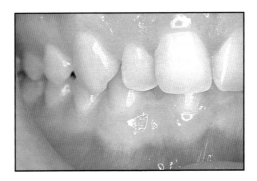

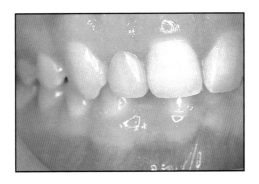

Tooth-colored plastic material was bonded onto this teenager's teeth to close the space between them. Alternative tooth-colored material was then used to recontour the lateral incisor, giving the illusion of straight teeth. The procedure is painless, fast, safe, and relatively inexpensive.

Protecting Your Child's Teeth at School and at Play

All along the way there will be hazards to your child's teeth from injury or accident. The toddler falls down in the course of learning to walk and run; the 3-year-old has blocks and swings and tricycles to contend with; and just as the older child begins to get a mouthful of permanent teeth, he or she goes in for a competitive sport and begins to use new tools and machines, such as bicycles and skateboards, for individual play. Safety education is important for dental health. Although your child's school probably emphasizes the same things as in the box below, your reinforcement helps.

Tips on Protecting Your Child's Teeth During Sports and Other Activities*

Sport/Activity	Safety tip
Football	Wear properly fitted mouth guard and helmet.
Baseball	Wear catcher's mask when receiving pitched balls.
Basketball	Wear a mouth guard, especially in rough games.
Boxing	Always wear a mouth guard.
Running games	Never trip or upset another player during play. Don't carry dangerous objects when you run.
Riding in cars	Be aware of sudden stops. Always wear a seat belt.
Swimming and diving	Use the ladder to climb out of the pool. Don't run or push when near a pool.
Tree climbing	Never climb a wet tree. Be sure of your footing.
Bicycling	Obey all traffic laws. Be careful in rainy weather. Wet roads and wet leaves make biking very dangerous.
Ice skating/Hockey	Don't push or trip other skaters. Wear a mouth guard when playing hockey.
Roller skating	Don't go too fast. Keep skates under control. Never "hitch" rides.
Swinging	Remain seated. Don't jump from or walk under a moving swing.
Sledding	Watch out for trees and other obstacles in your path.
Skateboarding	Apply nonskid tape to top of skateboard. Avoid busy streets and sidewalks. Avoid slopes—look for a flat surface.
Drinking from fountains	Don't startle your friends by speaking to them or touching them while they drink from a fountain. A quick movement or a slip could cause an accident.

*Adapted from the Detroit District Dental Society.

Teeth and Teenagers

There comes a time in the lives of parents when they look at their children and wonder, "Where did they come from — these strange, tall children, living in our home like boarders who don't pay rent and can't be evicted? Can these be the same children who 12 years ago were so charming and bright?" When we welcomed these babies with open arms, did we really understand that they would someday turn into teenagers?

It's hard for teenagers to find a dentist they can trust. Until they have the security of knowing where they are themselves, teenagers find dentists psychologically threatening. Their reluctance to have their mouths "invaded" is a displaced sexual fear.

I feel that the best way to reach teenage patients is to try to establish and maintain a strong personal relationship with them. Speak to your teenagers maturely and honestly. Tell them that it will make you happy and make them happy if they take care of their teeth.

There's not a teenager alive who is not thinking about sex — how they appear to others, how their smile looks, how their breath smells. Self-concepts and esthetics are strong motivators during the teenage years.

Get across to your teenager some positive message: "It makes you look brighter . . . Your smile looks good . . . It brightens up your face." These are encouraging words for teenagers.

Young people are not, as a rule, future-oriented; it does little good to talk to them about dental troubles they may face in their 20s and 30s.

As a dentist, I prefer to talk to a teenager without a parent around. I say, "Look, it's up to you. Your mother and your father have nothing to do with it anymore. You take care of your teeth or you don't. You know what's going on in your mouth. It's something you have to take care of for yourself."

The teenager also needs consistent and constant home and peer pressure. I know that parents don't like to hear this, but if Mom and Dad don't set a good example — if they are not committed to a self-care routine themselves — the child knows it and thinks of the parents as hypocritical. Advice and warnings then don't have any effect.

Young people are not, as a rule, future-oriented; it does little good to talk to them about dental troubles they may face in their 20s and 30s.

Bad Breath and Bleeding Gums

A boy or girl of 13 can understand scientifically that the odor from his or her mouth is from gas given off by the activity of the bacteria that live there. It is not caused by food sitting around in the mouth for too long. It is gas—hydrogen sulfide—the same gas that comes out of sewers. The only way to get rid of it is by daily cleaning.

It's ironic that just when teenagers become more aware of their looks, they become more careless of their diet and oral hygiene. Teenagers will try candy mints, chewing gum, mouthwashes, and other advertised products to sweeten their breath, and will neglect the one sure thing: thorough brushing and flossing. To show them what they're actually doing with their cleaning routine, suggest that they use a plaque-disclosing tablet once a week (see page 92).

The search for movie-star teeth may lead to the use of an abrasive toothpaste or one containing strong bleaches. Try to steer your teenagers away from these products without making them feel foolish.

Teenagers sometimes experience tender, bleeding gums, and their first thought is to stay away from the troublesome area. Actually, the very opposite treatment is called for; the more they brush and floss, the sooner the condition will clear up.

It's ironic that just when teenagers become more aware of their looks, they become more careless of their diet and oral hygiene.

Smoking

The teen years are a time of experimentation. This may lead to smoking, a habit that affects the teeth, palate, tongue, gums, lips, and throat, not to mention the total health of an individual. We know this now to be a scientific fact. It is a responsibility for all of us to dissuade teenagers from beginning to smoke. Again, be factual and forthright with your child: smokers have more gum disease, more oral cancer, stained teeth, bad breath, and deadened palates.

Teenage Orthodontics

The teen years are not too late for orthodontics. If your child has a problem in occlusion, orthodontics can correct it. But in the teen years it will be more important than ever that orthodontic treatment be accompanied by careful cleaning, daily fluoride, and snacking in moderation.

Wisdom Teeth

Wisdom teeth—actually, the third molars—usually come into the mouth in the late teens. Often a wisdom tooth is *impacted*—wedged against the molar in front of it—and must be removed. X-rays show the dentist whether the third molars are erupting in the right position and whether there is going to be room for these last molars in the dental arch.

Not all third molars have to be removed. Most discomfort comes from poor oral hygiene; third molars are difficult teeth to clean. If you'd like your teenager to be able to retain those teeth, having him or her use a water-irrigating device and thorough brushing may do the job.

Teenage Diets

Some teenagers eat the worst food imaginable, and the reason is not poverty. The potato chip and soft drink diet many teenagers become addicted to can be blamed on numerous elements. Many families no longer eat meals together as the children grow older, and children are allowed to raid the refrigerator and forage for themselves. Teenagers develop food fads and food preferences that limit their diets. They eat what their friends at the corner snack bar eat. Lots of carbohydrates are consumed in an effort to provide quick energy for sports and other strenuous activities and to face situations of emotional stress.

Not only do teenagers eat non-nutritious food, but they eat many times a day, a habit that feeds the bacteria as well as the teenager. Studies show that the average teenager eats nine times a day—usually snack foods. Snacks are a way of life for many teenagers; they become part of their social pattern.

All of this can add up to dental decay. Even if careful diet and regular dental care were part of early childhood, the effects can be wiped out by neglect and bad habits during the adolescent years.

So much is going on in the lives of these young people—physical, emotional, and social changes—that much of the resulting stress shows up in their general health, specifically in the teeth. Let's not give up our ambition—good teeth for our children's lifetime—at this vulnerable time in their lives. Try to encourage your teenager to snack in moderation and, above all, to brush twice daily with a fluoride toothpaste.

Bulimia

Bulimia, an eating disorder that is not uncommon among teenaged girls and sometimes boys, usually involves binge eating followed by purging—sometimes accomplished by use of a laxative, but more often by induced vomiting.

Often, the first person to detect this condition is the teenager's dentist. The tip-off is an odd kind of cavity on the tongue side of the front teeth; dentists generally recognize this as a sign that the patient is routinely inducing vomiting in an effort to control his/her weight.

The first step in treating the disorder is to have a candid discussion with the patient to explain how serious bulimia is; it can have a ruinous effect on the teeth and endanger the teenager's overall health. The patient's parents and physician should also be aware of the disorder, which in some cases may require counseling.

To minimize the dental consequences of bulimia, patients should add a daily fluoride mouthrinse to their oral hygiene routine.

REPORT CARD—3 YEARS

Look for these characteristics in your 3-year-old. If you can't answer "yes" to these questions, or if you have trouble completing this form, look back at Chapter 2 for more information or ask someone in your dentist's office to help you. See page 38 for the best way to examine your child's mouth; remember to use a good light.

Soft Tissues (Tongue, Lips, Cheeks, Gums)   Yes   No

Can your child stick the tip of his/her tongue completely out of the mouth?

Can your child swallow with the teeth together—without the tongue pushing through each time?

Are upper and lower lips the same size?

Is the lower lip free of chapping and cracking?

Is there a clear distinction between the lip and the skin of the face?

When you look inside the cheeks, are the entrances to the parotid glands even in size and not swollen? (The parotid glands, the major salivary glands, are marked by a little flap of skin inside the cheek, one on either side of the mouth.)

Is the color inside the cheeks even throughout?

Are gum tissues the same color, top and bottom? Front to back?

Are gums free of pimples? Swelling? (There should be no swelling, as no teeth are coming through just now.)

Hard Tissues (Teeth)

Number

Are there 20 teeth? Do you find 10 up and 10 down?

Are there the same number of teeth on either side of the midline?

Are the teeth on either side of the midline the same shape?

Bite

When your child closes the mouth, do the top teeth bite over the bottom teeth?

Do all the teeth come in contact when the jaw is closed?

Are the teeth spaced out, not crowded?

Color

Are the teeth milky white?

Are the teeth an even color from tips to gumline?

Are the top, bottom, front, and back teeth all the same color?

Do any stains and colors come off easily with a toothbrush?

Hygiene

Are the teeth clean?

Does the mouth have a clean, sweet odor?

Check for bad habits (see *Bad Habit "Checkup"* on page 46).

Are you brushing your child's teeth twice a day with an ADA-approved fluoride toothpaste?

Has your child seen a dentist for a checkup in the last 6 months?

Are you happy with your child's smile?

REPORT CARD—6 YEARS

Look for these characteristics in your 6-year-old. If you can't answer "yes" to these questions, or if you have trouble completing this form, look back at Chapter 2 for more information or ask someone in your dentist's office to help you. See page 38 for the best way to examine your child's mouth; remember to use a good light.

Soft Tissues (Tongue, Lips, Cheeks, Gums)   Yes   No

Is the tongue free of a white coating?

Can your child swallow with the teeth together—without the tongue pushing through each time?

Are upper and lower lips the same size?

Is the lower lip free of chapping and cracking?

Is there a clear distinction between the lip and the skin of the face?

When you look inside the cheeks, are the entrances to the parotid glands even in size and not swollen?

Is the color inside the cheeks even throughout?

Are gum tissues the same color, top and bottom? Front to back? Are gums free of pimples?

Is the tissue between the teeth firm, or loose and puffy? If you press it with your fingertip, does it bleed? (It shouldn't.)

Hard Tissues (Teeth)

Number

How many teeth are there? Are the front top or bottom teeth becoming loose? Have the permanent molars started to come in? Remember, they come in *behind*, not under, the primary molars.

Bite

When your child closes the mouth, do the top teeth bite over the bottom teeth?

Do all the teeth come in contact when the jaw is closed?

Are the teeth spaced out, not crowded?

Are you and your child pleased with the appearance of the teeth?

Do you have any concerns about possible malocclusion? If so, consult your child's dentist.

Have sealants been applied to the chewing surfaces and pits and fissures of your child's teeth?

Color

Are the teeth milky white?

Are the teeth an even color from tips to gumline?

Are the top, bottom, front, and back teeth all the same color?

Do any stains and colors come off easily with a toothbrush?

Hygiene

Are the teeth clean?

Does the mouth have a clean, sweet odor?

Check for bad habits (see *Bad Habit "Checkup"* on page 46).

Does your child brush twice daily with an ADA-approved fluoride toothpaste?

Does your child use disclosing tablets?

Has your child seen a dentist for a checkup in the last 6 months?

REPORT CARD—9 YEARS

Look for these characteristics in your 9-year-old. If you can't answer "yes" to these questions, or if you have trouble completing this form, look back at Chapter 2 for more information or ask someone in your dentist's office to help you. See page 38 for the best way to examine your child's mouth; remember to use a good light.

Soft Tissues (Tongue, Lips, Cheeks, Gums)   Yes   No

Is the tongue free of a white coating?

Can your child swallow with the teeth together—without the tongue pushing through each time?

Are upper and lower lips the same size?

Is the lower lip free of chapping and cracking?

Is there a clear distinction between the lip and the skin of the face?

When you look inside the cheeks, are the entrances to the parotid glands even in size and not swollen?

Is the color inside the cheeks even throughout?

Are gum tissues the same color, top and bottom? Front to back? Are gums free of pimples? Push the tongue aside and check the tongue side of the gum for abscesses.

Is the tissue between the teeth firm, or loose and puffy? If you press it with your fingertip, does it bleed? (It shouldn't.)

Hard Tissues (Teeth)

Number

How many teeth are there? There should now be at least four front permanent teeth in the upper and lower jaws, and four permanent molars, two up and two down.

Bite

When your child closes the mouth, do the top teeth bite over the bottom teeth?

Do all the teeth come in contact when the jaw is closed?

Are the teeth spaced out, not crowded?

Are the remaining primary molars worn down—is there any sign of grinding *(bruxism)*?

Are all the teeth at the same height in the jaw?

Are you and your child pleased with the appearance of the teeth?

Do you have any concerns about possible malocclusion? If so, consult your child's dentist.

Color

The permanent teeth are a shade darker than the primary teeth; are the new permanent teeth ivory colored and evenly shaded throughout?

Are the top, bottom, front, and back teeth all the same color?

Do any stains and colors come off easily with a toothbrush?

Hygiene

Are the teeth clean?

Does the mouth have a clean, sweet odor?

Does your child floss daily, in addition to brushing twice a day with an ADA-approved fluoride toothpaste?

Does your child use disclosing tablets?

Does your child have two toothbrushes? (It takes a day for one to dry out.)

Has your child had a new toothbrush in the last 6 months?

Has your child seen a dentist for a checkup in the last 6 months?

REPORT CARD—12 YEARS

Look for these characteristics in your 12-year-old. If you can't answer "yes" to these questions, or if you have trouble completing this form, look back at Chapter 2 for more information or ask someone in your dentist's office to help you. See page 38 for the best way to examine your child's mouth; remember to use a good light.

Soft Tissues (Tongue, Lips, Cheeks, Gums)

	Yes	No
Is the tongue free of a white coating?		
Can your child swallow with the teeth together—without the tongue pushing through each time?		
Are upper and lower lips the same size?		
Is the lower lip free of chapping and cracking?		
Is there a clear distinction between the lip and the skin of the face?		
When you look inside the cheeks, are the entrances to the parotid glands even in size and not swollen?		
Is the color inside the cheeks even throughout?		
Are gum tissues the same color, top and bottom? Front to back? Are gums free of pimples? Push the tongue aside and check the tongue side of the gum for abscesses.		
Is the tissue between the teeth firm, or loose and puffy? If you press it with your fingertip, does it bleed? (It shouldn't.)		

Hard Tissues (Teeth)

Number

How many permanent teeth are there? How many primary teeth? Most of the remaining primary teeth should be getting loose.		
Are there an even number of teeth on either side of the midline?		
The upper canines (the pointed teeth) should be coming into the mouth.		

Bite

When your child closes the mouth, do the top teeth bite over the bottom teeth?		
Do all the teeth come in contact when the jaw is closed?		
Do the teeth in front look long? When your child fails to brush, the gum can recede, creating a "long-toothed" look.		
Are you and your child pleased with the appearance of the teeth?		
Do you have any concerns about possible malocclusion? If so, consult your child's dentist.		

Color

The permanent teeth are a shade darker than the primary teeth; are the new permanent teeth ivory colored and evenly shaded throughout?		
Are the top, bottom, front, and back teeth all the same color?		
Do any stains and colors come off easily with a toothbrush?		

Hygiene

Are the teeth clean?		
Does the mouth have a clean, sweet odor?		
Does your child floss daily, in addition to brushing twice a day with an ADA-approved fluoride toothpaste?		
Does your child use disclosing tablets once a week?		
Does your child have two toothbrushes? (It takes a day for one to dry out.)		
Has your child had a new toothbrush in the last 6 months?		
Has your child seen a dentist for a checkup in the last 6 months?		

The Amazing Tooth

How a Tooth Begins

At birth, most of the primary teeth have begun to mineralize, and near them within the jaw the permanent teeth are forming.

Teeth are formed primarily from calcium and phosphate, which are taken from the bloodstream of the mother. She has incorporated these elements into her diet. Vitamin D and thyroid and growth hormones also play a part in the process. When the metabolic factors are normal, the manufacture of the teeth proceeds automatically, and the enamel and dentin crystals are healthy. If the metabolism is not normal, the crystals will mineralize imperfectly.

Although a pregnant mother's diet will affect the whole child, the developing teeth appear to be affected most by an imbalance of calcium and phosphorous salts in the bloodstream. An imbalance in these salts occurs most often from a high fever or a viral infection, not from a nutritional deficiency.

During tooth formation, the enamel crown forms from different centers on each tooth. Then these centers flow into each other and fuse together. The planes in which they fuse are the grooves and lines you see on the biting surface of molars.

Sometimes the centers don't fuse completely. This leaves a minute opening in the tooth—just big enough for bacteria to fit in. These spaces are called "pits" and "fissures"; a dentist can detect these by moving an explorer (pick) over the surface of the tooth.

The Parts of a Tooth

Let's take a look at a tooth—any tooth will do. The part you can see is the *crown*; the part that disappears into and is surrounded by the gum is called the *neck*; and the part you can't see, buried in the bony socket of the jaw and firmly anchored there by soft connecting tissues, is the *root*.

What a Tooth Is Made of

Enamel

The crown—the visible portion of the tooth—is covered with enamel, the hardest tissue in the body and one of the hardest natural substances known.

Enamel is composed of small crystals of calcium and phosphate precipitated in a fine matrix of strong protein fibers. Enamel has to be quite hard to do the job it is intended to do. First, it has to be resistant to acids, enzymes, and other corrosive substances found in the mouth. And it must protect the more sensitive tissues in the inner part of the tooth. The biting force of chewing can exert 50 to 100 pounds of pressure between the front teeth and 150 to 200 pounds between the teeth in the back! The enamel must absorb—and protect the dentin and pulp from—this impact.

Enamel is a crystal, and in the mouth it picks up and incorporates various minerals that make it harder. The longer enamel stays in a human's mouth, the harder it gets. That's probably one of the reasons that people over 20 get few cavities.

Enamel is also a unique crystal in that it can maintain its hardness over a wide range of temperature changes. It doesn't crack if you eat ice cream and then drink hot coffee.

Dentin

Dentin is the yellowish, bonelike tissue that lies just under the enamel. It is not as hard as enamel (which is why it needs the enamel to protect it), but is made of essentially the same materials—calcium salts and phosphate embedded in a strong network of protein fibers. Dentin forms the bulk of the tooth; the amount of dentin in a tooth determines its size and shape. Fibers from the pulp extend in small canals into the dentin and nourish it. If a cavity progresses toward the center of the tooth, the dentin cells in the pulp lay down a layer of protective dentin. Unfor-

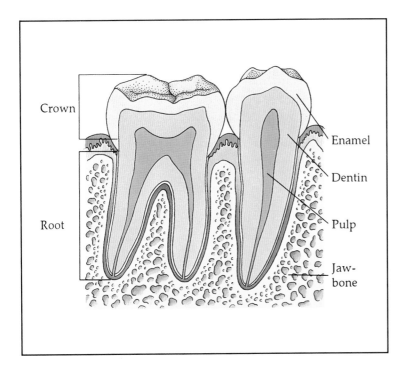

Parts of the teeth and supporting structure.

tunately, this is only a temporary defense, for if left alone, the decay progresses faster than the dentin is laid down, the pulp is invaded, and the tooth loses the battle.

Pulp

When your child has a toothache, the pulp is the part of the tooth that is sending the message. Dental pulp is the soft tissue that fills the chamber at the center of the tooth and the canals that extend down the roots of the tooth. The soft tissue here contains nerves and blood cells, and it is the source of the dentin's nutrition and the tooth's communication with the rest of the body. Pain is no fun, but it is the necessary signal to summon defense against caries, trauma, and infection. When the nerves in the pulp begin to signal, it's important to pay attention, for infection can and often does spread from a tooth to the rest of the body. Understanding this is important in handling a toothache emergency.

Cementum

Just as the hard enamel laminates and protects the crown (visible portion) of the tooth, the cementum—a thin, bone-like tissue—covers and protects the tooth root below the gums. It is not as hard as enamel and is less resistant to wear, as older people with receding gums too often find out. It forms fibers that, with other fibers formed by the bone, anchor the tooth to the bony socket and hold it in place.

The root makes up about two thirds of the total length of the tooth. The root is connected to the jawbone by special fibers that stretch like strips of elastic from the cementum covering to the bone that lines the tooth socket. These are called *periodontal fibers*, or *ligaments*, and running through them are the blood vessels that supply nutrition to the cementum. When dentists extract a tooth, they are not breaking bone; they are just separating the fiber that attaches the tooth to the bone. If teeth were actually part of the jaw, we couldn't remove a tooth without damaging the jawbone.

True or False?

"My children need lots of dental work because they had soft teeth to begin with."

False. All teeth are hard. As a matter of fact, tooth enamel is one of the hardest natural substances there is (diamonds are the hardest). Tooth enamel is much harder than iron, gold, or porcelain. Some teeth are more susceptible to decay than others, but it is never because the teeth are "soft." It is because they mineralized imperfectly or were not cared for after they came into the mouth.

There are two kinds of toothache generally seen in children, and understanding what causes both will make you better prepared to give first aid.

1. Toothaches That Occur During or After Eating

First is the kind of toothache that occurs while the child is eating or within a half hour or so after a meal or snack. The child will complain of sharp pain in the tooth. The food is in a cavity, feeding the bacteria living at the base of the cavity; the bacteria are producing acid that is seeping through the bottom of the tooth, reaching the nerve of the tooth and causing intense pain.

Put your child down, with his or her head in the examining position (see page 38) in your lap, and find out which tooth is painful. Take a toothbrush or toothpick and clean the tooth aggressively. If you are able to clean out all the food and bacteria this way, try to place a tiny piece of cotton in the hole, then in about 15 minutes the toothache will disappear. By all means, get your child to a dentist right away. Don't wait for another toothache. Decay progresses rapidly in a child's tooth.

2. Toothaches That Won't Go Away

The second type of toothache usually occurs at night and doesn't go away within an hour. The tooth is extremely sensitive to touch or to biting down, and the pain may be accompanied by a swollen area around the tooth or a warm, swollen jaw and face.

When this happens, it means that decay has progressed and the nerve inside the tooth has died and become infected and abscessed. This is a much more difficult kind of pain to relieve at home. Again, cleaning the tooth quite vigorously is the best thing you can do. See if you can open up the cavity and get out all the food.

An over-the-counter analgesic such as acetaminophen (swallowed, not held against the tooth) will relieve pain. Consult your dentist, pediatrician, or pharmacist about dosage. But the only real relief will be provided by a dentist, who will remove the tooth or make an opening in the tooth to allow gases and infection to escape.

If there is severe swelling and pain and you can't get to a dentist but can reach someone who can prescribe an antibiotic, this will help control the infection until a dentist can treat the tooth, which you should certainly arrange to have done as soon as possible.

As in most acute infections, the pain disappears after a few days. The gas breaks through the gum and bone and escapes. The pain is gone, but the infection remains.

You may see a gum boil when you examine a child's mouth after a toothache subsides. Check the sides of all the teeth to see if there is a pimple along the gum near a decayed tooth. This is the pathway along which gas and pus escape. The child is constantly swallowing infectious matter, which lowers resistance to other disease. Be sure that the child sees a dentist as soon as possible.

The Environment of the Teeth

The environment the teeth find themselves in is an active one. The taste buds—those busy cells that tell us what we like and what we don't like—are located here, and so are the salivary glands. Here are the lips, tongue, cheeks, and muscles of the jaw—the forces that are always pushing, pressing, moistening, and exerting environmental stress on the teeth.

... teeth can't tell the difference between hot and cold.

Teeth are remarkable. They can detect a fine grit between them. Their ability to sense size resides in little pressure receptors in the periodontal fiber, not in the teeth themselves. It is interesting that teeth can't tell the difference between hot and cold. When a child bites into ice cream or drinks hot soup, the teeth register not hot or cold, just pain. It's the lips and tongue that have the temperature receptors.

Supporting Structures

Fibers anchor the tooth's root to the jawbone. The alveolar bone is the bony portion of the upper and lower jaws that surrounds and supports the roots of the teeth and the gingiva, or gums. The health and integrity of these tissues are vitally important to the tooth. A sound, cavity-free tooth is only as secure as the structures that hold and support it.

The gums are a good diagnostic tool in detecting vitamin deficiencies because they react early. The gums are also susceptible to other problems, particularly those caused by the buildup of hard, razor-sharp deposits of tartar (*calculus*) along the gum line. The gums move away from the bacteria that live on the tartar and, in so doing, move away from the tooth, allowing pockets to form, where food particles and bacteria are caught. Infection that begins here can damage the gums, beginning with inflammation and tiny tears in the surface tissue. The first sign of infection you may notice is bleeding of the gums when the teeth are brushed.

The periodontal ligament is also susceptible to infection. Inflammation caused by toxins from the bacteria in the plaque around the neck of the tooth will loosen the periodontal attachment. Eventually, infection will reach the alveolar bone.

Gum diseases are often found in older teenagers and adults but are sometimes diagnosed in children.

An interesting fact is that in a healthy mouth the response to hard use of all of these supporting structures—the gums, periodontal ligament, and alveolar bone—is their strengthening. For instance, the stress of chewing tough foods and the stress of vigorous brushing, shared evenly by the teeth, make the gums, ligaments, and bone stronger, and keep them in better tone. On the other hand, if an area of the mouth gets no use—because of missing teeth or because a malocclusion or a cavity discourages chewing in that area—then the tissues lose tone, the ligaments lose strength and elasticity, and the underlying alveolar bone may actually break down, decalcify, and be lost.

Saliva: The "Bloodstream" of the Teeth

It may come as a surprise to you that teeth are not static: they continually lose small amounts of mineral and take up minerals to replace the loss. And just as the bloodstream moves essential nutrients throughout the body, so the saliva brings mineral building-blocks into contact with the teeth.

The salivary glands are located in the cheeks and in the floor of the mouth. When you are looking at your baby's mouth, familiarizing yourself with the "inside" as well as the "outside," locate and look at the openings of the parotid salivary glands in the cheeks so you won't be startled by them later and wonder what they are. They are small flaps of tissue, on the inside of both cheeks, that indicate the openings of the major salivary glands.

Saliva is a remarkable substance that performs several useful jobs in the mouth. Like a "liquid enamel," saliva is super-saturated with calcium and phosphate—the basic minerals that make up tooth enamel. Fluoride, from dietary and topical sources, is also present in the saliva. Together, these three elements work continually to shore up tooth enamel. When the essential ingredients are all present in the mouth, small breaches in the tooth caused by the activity of caries bacteria can actually "heal" before any serious damage is done.

This is why it's so important to regularly replenish the "fluoride reservoir" in the mouth. (See Chapter 5 for more

True or False?

"When a youngster's gums bleed, just leave them alone. They will heal by themselves."

False. Most often it's the food and bacteria that collect at the spot where the gums meet the teeth that are causing the trouble. Brush more effectively. In two or three days, the gums will usually toughen up and won't bleed so readily. They will continue to stay well unless you again fail to brush them properly.

about that.) Each time you brush with a fluoride toothpaste or drink a glass of fluoridated water, for instance, some of the fluoride stays in your mouth for several hours, stored in the saliva, on the teeth, and in the soft tissues—even in plaque. That stored fluoride is readily available when and where it's needed to counteract an acid challenge from decay-causing bacteria.

Another remarkable property of saliva is its buffering capacity, that is, its ability to neutralize acid. We know that acid is formed in the mouth when food debris is broken down by bacteria. This acid, held against the tooth in plaque, destroys the enamel and makes decay possible. The particular chemical makeup of saliva enables it to neutralize these acids. What's more, saliva even seems to have antimicrobial properties that help inhibit bacterial growth in the mouth.

There are some individuals who go through life without ever getting a cavity. Dental researchers are studying the saliva of these individuals in order to discover whether its composition holds the secret to their cavity-free state.

Saliva is noteworthy for its other important functions. A drop in the saliva output will trigger the sensation of thirst, reminding the body to take in more water and thus serving to regulate water balance. Saliva lubricates food, making chewing and swallowing easier. And it contains an enzyme that aids oral clearance of starchy foods that can promote tooth decay.

As air moves through the mouth, drying the teeth and the gum tissues, saliva remoistens them. Saliva also helps to wash the teeth free of food debris—but this doesn't mean you can give up your toothbrush. Nature needs all the help it can get.

Over the years we've learned so much about the positive effects of saliva in the mouth that many dentists now recommend sugarless chewing gum after a snack or meal to stimulate saliva at the precise time when it may do the most good, that is, when oral bacteria are most active.

. . . many dentists now recommend sugarless chewing gum after a snack or meal to stimulate saliva.

The Bacterial Population in Your Mouth

Also part of the teeth's environment are some 80 varieties of microorganisms—a fairly stable population in any-body's mouth. A recent important research discovery is that of these 80 or so different bacteria, only three or four are responsible for caries.* And even more interesting, only certain kinds attack certain areas of the tooth. In other words, the bacteria that make holes on the biting surface of a tooth are different from those that make holes at the gum line or on the side. These three or four bacteria have two things in common that make them susceptible to destruction. They all need time to organize into colonies on the teeth (plaque) and they need food to survive. This information gives us the keys to defensive dentistry.

As we have seen, the tooth in its environment is pushed around by the dynamic forces of moving muscles, washed in a bath of saliva, affected by extremes of temperature as we feed ourselves hot dogs and ice cream, and dried by the flow of air into and out of the lungs. The mouth is a busy crossroads of the body and important to our anatomy and to our psyche. We've had a close look at the tooth. Now let's take an in-depth look at its maintenance.

---

*Another important caries-research breakthrough of recent years shows that rats raised in a germ-free environment do not develop caries until rats with caries are introduced into the germ-free colony.

A Complete Guide to Clean Teeth

Tipping the Scale Toward No Decay

There is an interesting clinical phenomenon that I see as a pediatric dentist. Of two children in the same family, one may have a history of decay and the other may reach the age of 12 or 14 without having had a single cavity. People point to these two children and say, "They live in the same house, are given the same foods, have the same things happening to them. Why the difference? Does one have something in his genetic inheritance that blessed him with decay-resistant teeth?"

In my mind there is very little in heredity that bears on dental decay. The real difference between these two children is their habits. One may brush the teeth thoroughly; the other, halfheartedly. One may snack too frequently; the other less often. Differences like these may seem very slight, but they add up.

There are many factors that can cause dental breakdown, and it's not until the combination of accumulated factors reaches a certain point that the scale for one individual is tipped toward decay.

Teeth have a great resistance to decay. The best way to prevent decay is to understand all the factors that can tip the scales the wrong way, and then work toward lifting the factors you can control from the negative side of the scale, so that the scale is balanced on the side of prevention.

What are some of the factors that can tip the scale toward cavities? To understand them, you first must understand how cavities form.

The simplest way is to think of a tooth as a child's wooden block. In your mind, picture that block with a lump of clay stuck to it. The clay is plaque. And suspended in the clay are lots of tiny beads—bacteria. The clay "plaque" sticks to the block and holds bacteria against the block's surface.

What Is Plaque?

Plaque is a sticky, transparent film that clings tenaciously to the teeth and can hardly be seen. It forms all the time, 24 hours a day.

You may recognize plaque as the stuff you can scrape off your teeth with your fingernail. A milligram of plaque may contain as many as 200 to 500 million bacteria. In fact, bacteria cause plaque.

The bacteria that live on the teeth have a special problem: the tongue and lips, saliva, food, and drink all have the potential to sweep bacteria off the teeth and into the stomach. So in order to cling to the teeth, bacteria secrete a "bacterial glue" called dextran. This remarkable substance resists water, which explains why rinsing your mouth doesn't budge plaque.

In addition to providing a secure foothold for bacteria, dextran serves other purposes. It acts as a net to trap little bits of the food you eat, so the bacteria have convenient provisions. And when there is no food available, bacteria digest some of their own dextran to tide them over until your next meal.

The stuff we call plaque, then, is a conglomeration of bacteria, the sticky dextran they've secreted, and tiny bits of food trapped in it.

But it's even more complex. Plaque harbors a variety of

microorganisms. Those near the outside surface are bacteria that thrive in the presence of oxygen; those nearer the tooth surface are bacteria that flourish in the presence of carbon dioxide.

As these different bacteria digest foods, they secrete another by-product, organic acids. Trapped in the sticky substance, these acids are held in contact with the tooth. The result of prolonged exposure to acids is a net loss of mineral from the tooth. If the situation is allowed to progress, eventually a cavity will form directly under the plaque layer.

Cavities aren't the only consequence of poor oral hygiene. Much of the plaque forms at the gum line, where it can cause irritation, bleeding gums, and worse problems.

However, there is an interesting positive aspect to plaque: it has the ability to stockpile fluoride in the form of an acid-soluble crystal. When you eat carbohydrates (sugars or cooked starches), bacteria rapidly begin metabolizing and within seconds start producing measurable quantities of acid. But if there is fluoride stored in the plaque, the acid attack will dissolve the fluoride crystals and release fluoride precisely when and where it is needed to fight demineralization and promote remineralization.

Despite its fluoride-storing capabilities, plaque is not good for your teeth. That's why dentists emphasize removing plaque regularly. Brushing twice daily with a fluoride toothpaste and flossing once a day is a good policy.

Once plaque is removed, it takes about a day for the bacteria to regroup and rebuild their plaque community. After 2 days, when they are securely entrenched, they will resume producing enough acid to threaten the teeth and gums. If left undisturbed, plaque sometimes begins to harden and form tartar, which you can't scrape off with a toothbrush or a fingernail. The dentist or dental hygienist must remove tartar with special tools.

When you eat carbohydrates (sugars or cooked starches), bacteria rapidly begin metabolizing and within seconds start producing measurable quantities of acid.

Plaque and Tooth Decay

The first sign of tooth decay is a white spot on the surface of the tooth. (At this stage, decay can still be stopped and reversed.) This white spot shows where plaque acids are leaching minerals from the enamel. After a time, so much mineral is lost that a hole forms. As mineral loss continues, the soft inner part of the tooth is affected and the destructive process speeds up. Eventually, the decay reaches the nerve center. If you haven't had a warning pain before, you'll have it now. Result: at best, you'll need a redundant filling; at worst, you may require root canal treatment, or you might even lose the tooth.

Plaque and Periodontal Disease

Plaque also sets the stage for periodontal or gum disease. It begins when plaque creeps into the fold of tissue at the gum line, along the root of the tooth. Bacteria in the plaque may die off and mineralize, forming tartar. As plaque moves deeper into the gums, you'll notice inflammation, redness, and puffiness. The condition may worsen until the supporting tissues pull away; eventually, the tooth literally falls out.

Of course, that's a horror story for grown-ups. Adults suffer more from periodontal disease than from decay. However, gum problems are not limited to adults; almost everybody experiences some degree of gingivitis (inflammation of the gums) at one time or another. Bleeding gums are a symptom of infection.

Researchers have demonstrated that if a normal human subject completely ceases practicing oral hygiene, gingivitis will result within a couple of weeks. When oral hygiene and plaque-control methods are resumed, gingivitis clears up. It might be expected that if a person neglects oral hygiene indefinitely, he or she runs the risk of losing teeth and even the supporting bone. Experiments in this area have not been carried out because the end result, unlike gingivitis, is irreversible. A few days of thorough brushing will clear up gingivitis in a child. Don't worry if initially brushing makes the gums seem to bleed more.

How Can We Control Bacteria?

By now it should be clear that bacteria and the plaque they form can cause a lot of trouble in the mouth. Why can't we control them?

It would be ideal if we had a vaccine against the bacteria that cause dental cavities. But we don't, and it's doubtful that one will be developed soon.

Another futuristic solution would be a strain of "good bacteria" that we could put in our mouths to crowd out the cavity-causing bacteria. That's also not on the books yet.

Still another suggestion—one that has been tried with

laboratory animals for a long time—is to use antibiotics to cut down a broad range of organisms in the mouth. In these experiments, no matter what diet the laboratory animals are fed, they don't get dental caries—for a while. Unfortunately, new strains of antibiotic-resistant bacteria eventually evolve in the mouth. So much for that solution.

Plaque Control

Now for the good news: while we haven't conquered the oral bacteria problem, we can control it. If the formation of plaque is interrupted at least once every 24 hours, bacteria cannot produce enough acid to harm your teeth and gums.

This is one of the key concepts of preventive dentistry, and it grew out of the research on plaque. If you spend a few minutes daily brushing and flossing away plaque, you'll be taking the single most important step toward oral health. Only you can control the plaque in your mouth.

If the formation of plaque is interrupted at least once every 24 hours, bacteria cannot produce enough acid to harm your teeth and gums.

The Old Toothbrushing Technique

If you're of a "certain age," you may still be using an outmoded technique to clean your teeth. There is a newer approach than the old up-and-down or side-to-side vigorous scrubbing, and in case no one has demonstrated the technique to you, I'll take you through the basic steps so that you can teach it to your children. This method helps prevent cavities in children and gum disease in adults.

Remember the old advice, "Brush twice a day; see your dentist twice a year"? Good, but inadequate. The old brushing method was intended to polish teeth and remove food particles. The new way emphasizes plaque control.

The old brushing technique called for up-and-down strokes with a hard-bristle brush, and for dental floss used occasionally to remove a recalcitrant food particle. The new way removes the plaque, and flossing is a must.

The New Toothbrushing Technique

There are a number of acceptable toothbrushing methods that clean food debris from the teeth, but I want to suggest

The major dental complaint of adults is tooth sensitivity to hot and cold liquids. The cause of this problem is overly aggressive toothbrushing as a child and young adult. Twice-daily gentle brushing is sufficient to prevent tooth decay and maintain healthy gums!

one—a kind of soft-scrub method that children can handle—that will remove plaque.

To instruct your child, try the soft-scrub stroke on your child's hand. Place the brush in the child's palm and move the bristles forward about one-half inch, without actually displacing the head of the brush. Flexing the bristles is all that is necessary. You'll produce a kind of jiggling or vibrating movement. Try it on your own hand and you'll see what I mean. Now lighten the pressure, speed up the movements, and there you have the soft-scrub stroke.

This is the way we teach. However, I don't insist on every point. If a child is more comfortable or more adept at brushing in a different direction—even in circles—it's fine with me. Children most often miss the tongue side of the back molars and the cheek side of the upper molars.

A word of caution: excessive pressure over the years can wear away enamel. A soft brush and gentle pressure in its use are best.

How to Brush Your (and Your Child's) Teeth

1. Place the head of your toothbrush alongside your teeth, with the bristle tips angled against the gum line. Look at yourself in the mirror as you brush. I feel strongly that there should be a child-level mirror in every bathroom.

2. Move the brush back and forth with short strokes—about half a tooth wide. Use a gentle scrubbing motion, brushing one or two teeth at a time and then moving the brush on to the next couple of teeth.

3. Here is a way to brush the entire mouth systematically. Start with the last tooth and then move toward the front of the mouth brushing the outside surfaces. Still using the same short, back-and-forth strokes, brush the inside surfaces. Brush all four quarters of the mouth.

4. To brush the insides of the front teeth, hold the brush vertically, angle the bristles toward your gums, and use short up-and-down strokes.

5. Now, keeping the brush flat, brush the chewing surfaces of your teeth. Don't forget the pits and grooves on molars—it's sometimes hard to clean these surfaces. You can even clean your tongue with your toothbrush—makes your mouth feel fresher.

6. Rinse vigorously. Smile.

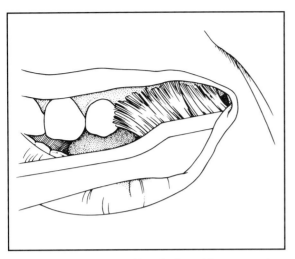

Place the head of the toothbrush alongside your teeth, with the bristle tips angled against the gum line.

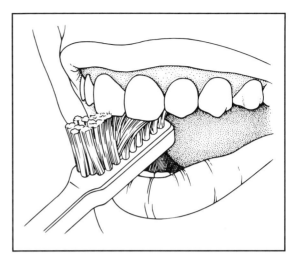

Brush the insides of the front teeth (upper and lower) with the front part of the toothbrush.

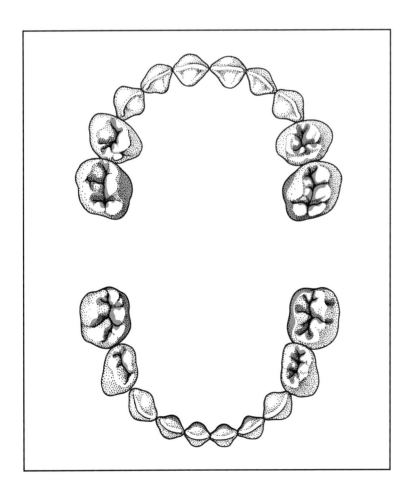

Areas shown in red are those most often missed by children when brushing.

Flossing is Easy—And Important

You may have used floss to dislodge bits of food caught between the teeth. Perhaps you never thought of it as a means for removing plaque, or what I call shining the adjacent sides of the teeth.

Even the best brush cannot completely remove plaque between the teeth and beneath the gum line. Flossing does remove plaque and debris from between the teeth and below the gum line—areas where decay often starts.

Young children may have difficulty managing a length of floss as described below. As an alternative, take a piece of floss about 12 or 14 inches long and knot the ends together so that the child has a circle with which to work. Or you can buy an easy-to-handle plastic floss holder at most drugstores.

One of the most important places for a youngster to floss is between the last two molars in each jaw. As the child grows older and the natural spaces between the teeth grow smaller, he or she can become as adept as you in the method outlined below.

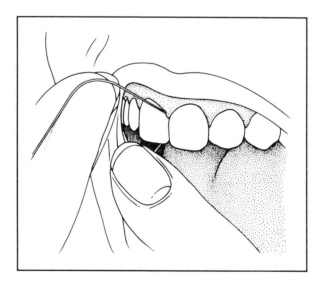

Use dental floss to clean the sides of your teeth. Floss goes under the gum line. It should be used to clean tooth surfaces on both sides of every space.

How to Floss Your Teeth

1. Break off about 18 inches of floss and wind most of it around one of your middle fingers. The middle finger of the opposite hand can take up the used floss as you work on your teeth.

2. Holding the floss taut (there should be no slack), keep one inch free and, with a gentle, sawing motion, slide it between your teeth. Don't be rough.

3. When it reaches the gum line, curve the floss in a "C" shape against a tooth, gently sliding it into the space between the gum and the tooth.

4. Holding the floss tightly against the tooth, scrape the floss up and down against the side of one tooth. Then curve it against the neighboring tooth and again scrape up and down. This will break up the plaque and remove the bacteria.

5. Think of your mouth as having four sections; floss one section at a time. Once you establish a regular pattern, you can do it without thinking and you won't miss any of your teeth.

Flossing is a skill that can be developed with a little practice. After you've flossed for a few days, you will find that it will take only a few minutes of your time. Flossing can be done anytime—while you're reading or watching television—but flossing at bedtime is best because it means a clean mouth throughout the nighttime hours. It will be 24 hours before plaque again reaches a critical plateau.

Brushing and flossing are the basic tools of plaque control. They are the easiest, best, least expensive ways to remove plaque from the teeth and gums.

The Right Toothbrush

Adopt a new attitude toward your old friend the toothbrush. It's not just something to make your teeth attractive, it's a weapon for removing food and attacking plaque. The right brush for the method of toothbrushing just described has a straight handle, soft bristles, a flat brushing surface, at least three rows of bristles, and a small head.

A soft nylon brush with double-rounded, small bristles is good. The tufts of the bristles should all be the same length. The head of the brush should be small enough so that children can reach all the teeth in their mouth, at the gum line as well as the grooved molar surfaces.

Everybody should (need I say it?) use only his or her own toothbrush and replace it promptly when it begins to wear out (about every 4 months). Store it in a place where it will dry quickly and won't touch other brushes. Have two toothbrushes on hand and use them alternately, and maybe even have one more toothbrush in reserve in case the bristles of your old brush begin to look frayed, limp, and loose.

It takes a day for a nylon toothbrush to dry out. If a child is using the same brush every day, it gets too soft to do an adequate job. Another piece of advice: After an illness have your child get a new toothbrush. Colds that persist all winter may be caused by toothbrushes harboring bacteria that keep reinfecting your child.

Colds that persist all winter may be caused by toothbrushes harboring bacteria that keep reinfecting your child.

Electric Toothbrushes

The same points apply to the brushing head of an electric toothbrush. A powered brush, used properly, can be effective, and can be especially helpful for children with certain disabilities. But a person who brushes carelessly with a regular toothbrush will do the same with an electric device.

Electric toothbrushes are more efficient than manual toothbrushes. However, they have major problems. Like other "labor saving" electric devices stored in odd corners of the bathroom and kitchen, electric toothbrushes get to be too much trouble to get out, assemble, and use every day. Then, too, parents buy electric toothbrushes in the hope that they will encourage children to brush. The novelty works only for a while—as with any new toy.

I would buy an electric brush only for the child who has already developed the habit of cleaning his or her teeth every day. Otherwise, it will soon be available for cleaning the algae off the sides of fish tanks or for shining shoes.

Mouthwashes

Ordinary mouthwashes temporarily freshen breath and sweeten the mouth but do not remove plaque and cannot prevent dental disease. In fact, their use may mask a condition that needs professional attention.

Fluoride mouthrinses, on the other hand, bring fluoride in contact with the teeth. They should be used after brushing.

Water-Irrigating Devices

Oral-irrigating devices that shoot small jets of water between and around teeth will flush out loose debris and can be especially helpful to children wearing braces, teenagers with wisdom teeth, and older people with bridgework. The jets of water feel good. The devices don't, however, remove plaque. They're not a substitute for brushing. Plaque is too tenacious.

Interdental Devices

Besides dental floss, other interdental devices are available. They include rubber-tipped probes; toothpick-like instruments; and wooden, plastic, and quill devices. Don't give these to your child. They are of questionable value in removing plaque from youngsters' teeth and can scratch and injure gum tissue.

While we are taking a look at misconceptions about plaque removal, let me list some other things that have been shown not to be effective substitutes for brushing and flossing: eating crisp food, rinsing the mouth with water, and chewing gum.

What Toothpaste Is Best?

Any fluoride-containing toothpaste recognized by the American Dental Association as being effective in reducing tooth decay is recommended. Toothpastes have a number of advantages:

- They bring fluoride in contact with the tooth surface. The more times and the more ways fluoride is brought in contact with a tooth, the stronger that tooth will be and the more resistant to decay.
- Toothpastes contain a detergent material that helps the brush sweep away some of the debris found on teeth.
- Toothpastes have a pleasant taste and leave your mouth feeling refreshed after you've brushed.

You might ask, "If the water supply is fluoridated, is it really that beneficial to use a fluoride toothpaste?" Yes—*definitely*. The uptake of fluoride is a surface phenomenon. Research shows that topical (surface) fluoride provides a benefit in addition to that which comes from fluoride in your drinking water.

"If the water supply is fluoridated, is it really that beneficial to use a fluoride toothpaste?" Yes—definitely.

How Much Toothpaste Should You Use?

While I'm on the subject of toothpaste, I want to clarify something. For years, toothpaste commercials have fondly shown Mom, Dad, Junior, and Sis gleefully squeezing generous ribbons of toothpaste on to their toothbrushes. And why not? The manufacturers want us to buy toothpaste—lots of it. But the truth is, all anyone really needs to do a good cleaning job is a pea-sized dab of toothpaste. At that rate, you'll be amazed how far a tube of toothpaste can last.

Use Caution With Child-Appealing, Flavored Toothpastes

Make sure your children understand that toothpaste is not a food or a treat and it should not be swallowed.

In recent years, toothpaste marketing has taken on a new and potentially problematic twist: manufacturers are selling toothpaste in new, child-appealing flavors that are literally good enough to eat. That's the problem: I know of cases where children *are* eating such flavorful toothpastes. If you decide to buy these products, use extra caution. Make sure your children understand that toothpaste is not a food or a treat and it should not be swallowed. Younger children who can't understand that sort of information must be closely supervised while they brush.

Try an Experiment With Disclosing Tablets

How can you tell when your child's teeth are really clean? You can locate the plaque on teeth by using disclosing tablets or liquids that temporarily stain the plaque with harmless vegetable dyes. The color will disappear gradually but completely. Be sure to explain the experiment to a child carefully beforehand; your child will be interested in the process. The tablets are inexpensive and can be purchased at any drugstore, or perhaps your dentist will give you some. I find disclosing tablets to be a good teaching device. A small piece of one tablet is adequate for most children.

Check out your own mouth, along with those of your children. Chew a tablet for 30 seconds without swallowing. Now rinse your mouth out with water. Swish the liquid all around the teeth, then spit. Examine your teeth in a good source of light so that you can see their inner and outer surfaces. Study the pattern of plaque accumulation in your mouth. Every mouth is different. There is considerable individual variation in the amount of plaque formed and in its distribution in different parts of the mouth.

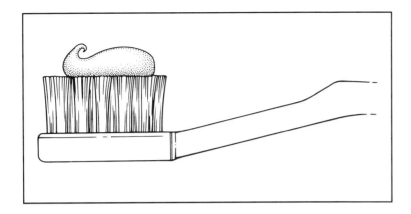

A small dab of toothpaste is all that is needed to do a good cleaning job.

You'll probably see that the areas with the darkest stains are between the teeth, along the gum line, on any roughened surface or crack, and on any area that is protected from lip, tongue, and cheek action by the tooth's shape or position. These will probably always be the places where you should concentrate your cleaning efforts. (See page 87 for the places children most often miss.)

It's a good idea to use a disclosing tablet periodically to see how well you are cleaning your teeth.

The "Buddy System"

When I was a child, my mother made a habit of checking up on me after my showers, looking behind my ears and under my arms to ensure that I was thoroughly clean. But I hated showering, so I would go into the bathroom, close the door, turn on the shower, and sit on the floor reading a comic book for a suitable period of time. Then, just before coming out to present myself for inspection, I'd dampen the areas behind my ears and under my arms.

I confide this information not to impress you with my cleverness, but to remind you that children don't always share our goals and objectives. You may care passionately about your child's oral hygiene; your child may not care a whit.

To complicate matters, children are also very resourceful. I wasn't the first kid to figure out how to get around a problem like showering, and I certainly wasn't the last.

I can't tell you how to make your child care about dental health. In fact, I'm of the opinion that you *can't* make a child care. So your best alternative is to monitor your family's toothbrushing and flossing routines.

For a child up to the age of 8 or so, the best insurance is supervised brushing—what I call the buddy system. A child who doesn't wash his or her face and hands can't get away with it very long—the evidence is pretty hard to conceal. But a child who doesn't brush his or her teeth very likely can fake it for a long time. A toothbrushing buddy can be an older brother or sister or a parent—someone who will make sure the job is done regularly and well. This adds to the control and accuracy of your child's cleaning program.

How to Protect the Tooth's Surface From Decay

The surface of the tooth is naturally hard and impermeable to the penetration of acid unless the acid remains for a long time. A tooth's surface is usually bathed with saliva, which, besides keeping the tooth moist, contains substances whose buffering effect neutralizes acids.

The tooth's surface can be made even stronger by incorporating fluoride into it. Enamel is a crystal structure composed of several elements. One of its molecules can be replaced with a harder mineral—fluoride—if it is present when the tooth is forming. If this substitution takes place, the crystal matrix of the tooth is all the more resistant to acid.

There are a number of ways to get fluoride. You can do it topically: a fluoride application at the dentist's office, a fluoride mouthrinse, fluoride toothpaste—even fluoridated water has a topical effect as it passes through the mouth. And you can take fluoride systemically by drinking fluoridated water or taking supplemental fluoride. See Chapter 5 for a complete discussion of fluoride.

Sealants

One way to combat plaque and acid on the teeth is to use sealants. A sealant is a coat of plastic material applied to the biting surface of the back teeth to help shield them from plaque and acid. The bacteria can make all the acid they want; the acid won't penetrate the sealant. Sealants for

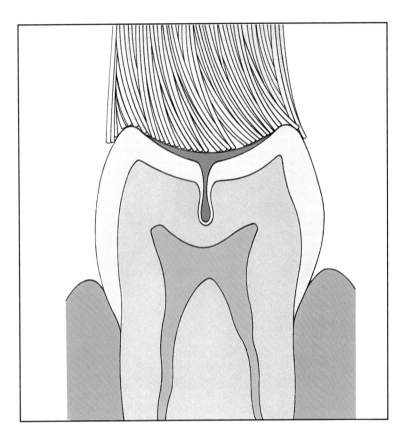

Tooth crevice filled with sealant (in blue). The tooth is protected from decay and the smooth biting surface makes cleaning easier.

tooth surfaces have been in use for about 20 years, especially for the biting surfaces of molars. Sealants for the entire tooth are under study.

Sealants have proven to be long-lasting and extremely effective in protecting vulnerable tooth surfaces from decay.

Contouring Teeth

Another technique that dentists have known for a long time but practice infrequently is reshaping the biting surfaces of the molars, grinding away the tiny nooks and crannies that tend to trap food particles and bacteria.

Contouring the teeth is actually just rushing nature a little bit—most people wear their molars down somewhat over the years anyway.

By reshaping the little hills and valleys of the molar surfaces, the dentist makes the tooth surface more saucerlike. A smoother surface discourages food accumulation and helps cut down on the formation of plaque.

The Best Ways to Help Your Child Avoid Tooth Decay

- Help your child practice good oral hygiene. Teeth should be brushed thoroughly (with supervision by a parent or other buddy) two times a day—after breakfast and before bedtime. The same is true for an infant: clean the teeth and gums at least twice daily.
- Make sure your child gets fluoride. Possible sources include drinking water, over-the-counter fluoride toothpastes and mouthrinses, and topical fluoride treatments applied by the dentist approximately every 6 months.
- Because most meals and snacks contain sugars or cooked starches, the more often your child eats, the more often he or she "feeds" decay-causing bacteria. Limit meals and snacks to a reasonable number.
- To discourage baby-bottle tooth decay, never let a child use a feeding bottle as a pacifier.
- Have your dentist apply protective sealant to the chewing surfaces of your child's teeth as early as possible.

The Fluoride Story

Fluoridation, the most effective and economical method of protecting the tooth against decay, is one of the greatest achievements in the history of public health. It ranks right along with vaccination, pasteurization, and chlorination—all public health measures that were controversial in their time.

A community that has decided to fluoridate its water has, in effect, decided to reduce dental disease in its children by 50% to 75%. Since fluoridation saves money as well as teeth, the cost of dental care in that community is reduced. Chicago, one of the first major cities to fluoridate its water (1956), saved more than $20 million in dental bills in the first 15 years of fluoridation, as tooth decay dropped by 50% among its school population.

Questions Commonly Asked About Fluoride

What is fluoride? What does it do? How is it used? How safe is it? Does it do adults any good? These are some of the questions people ask about fluoride. I am particularly interested in answering them because, as a young dental student in the late 1950s, I worked on the historic Kingston-Newburgh experiment. The story of fluoride is an intriguing tale, one of the best real detective stories. In 1901 a dentist who had just graduated and started his practice in Colorado Springs began puzzling over the fact that his young patients had brown stains and mottling on their teeth that he could not remove. "It's the water," local residents said. That was only a kind of folk wisdom, because today's sophisticated methods of chemical analysis had not been developed. There were lots of theories about the stain but no scientific explanation.

By communicating with dentists in other areas and working with the US Public Health Service, the young dentist eventually found that water was indeed the cause of the unsightly brown stain. The water in Colorado Springs—principally supplied from melted snow pouring down the mineral-bearing deposits on the slopes of Pikes Peak—contained a relatively high amount of dissolved fluoride.

As dentists began to focus on the cause of mottling—"Colorado Brown Stain," as the condition was sometimes called (*dental fluorosis* is the technical term)—they made another amazing discovery: the teeth of children with this degree of severe fluorosis also were remarkably resistant to decay. Could something that made teeth look bad also be good for them?

As more studies were performed, it was discovered that too much fluoride in water led to a cosmetically unacceptable degree of fluorosis, but just enough brought enormous benefits without perceptibly affecting the appearance of the teeth.

"Just enough" turned out to be one part fluoride to one million parts water (1 ppm). This was established in rigorous tests, such as the one in which I took part in Newburgh, a community in New York State that decided to fluoridate its water (to 1.1 ppm), while Kingston, a neighboring city with fluoride-deficient water (0.1 ppm), served as a control.

There was a constant downward trend in cavities in Newburgh's children, with the younger children showing the greatest benefits.

Very thorough medical comparisons were made—growth rates, tonsillectomy rates, skeletal maturation,

Fluoridated vs Nonfluoridated Water

Newburgh (fluoridated)	Kingston (nonfluoridated)
41% of the 5- and 6-year-olds had no cavities.	17% of the 5- and 6-year-olds had no cavities.
Mean annual cost for dental treatment at age 5 was $13.86.	Mean annual cost for dental treatment at age 5 was $33.73.
Mean annual cost for dental treatment at age 6 was $16.93.	Mean annual cost for dental treatment at age 6 was $40.78.

bone density—every test that could be thought of. The conclusion of long-term pediatric studies was that there was no indication of any effects, good or bad, from adjusting the level of fluoride in the drinking water—except for the reduction in cavities.

Let's look at another town's experience. Antigo, Wisconsin, after 11 years of fluoridating its water supply, for financial reasons reversed its decision and stopped. Within 6 years, the cavity rate in kindergartners had gone up 112%. The town changed its mind again and went back to fluoridated water.

A fluoridated water supply is extremely safe. How safe is extremely safe? There is nothing anywhere—in scientific literature, in test reports, in statistics, in the history of people who drank naturally fluoridated water long before some communities decided to add fluoride to their water supplies—to indicate or suggest that fluoride ever affected anything but the appearance of the teeth.

The list of organizations worldwide that endorse fluoridation is lengthy, everyone from the American Dental Association, the American Academy of Pediatric Dentistry, the American Academy of Pediatrics, and the American Association for Dental Research to the American Cancer Society, the American Institute of Nutrition, the American Medical Association, the American Osteopathic Association, and the US Public Health Service. And that's just a small sample of United States organizations that back fluoride!

While a lot of questions have been raised over the years by antifluoride groups, by and large, not one of them has had anything interesting or relevant to say. When analyzed, their arguments have much to do with attitudes that are antigovernmental and antiscientific, but little to do

Popular Misconceptions About Fluoridation

1. *Misconception:* Fluoride causes cancer.

   Fact: Epidemiologic studies comparing death rates from cancer show no significant differences between fluoridated and nonfluoridated communities.

2. *Misconception:* Fluoride causes kidney dysfunction.

   Fact: Studies show no differences in kidney function rates among residents of cities with varying amounts of fluoride in their drinking water.

3. *Misconception:* Fluoride causes heart disease.

   Fact: Long-term fluoridation does not adversely affect cardiovascular disease mortality rates.

4. *Misconception:* Fluoride causes allergies.

   Fact: The fluoride levels used in water supplies are too low to cause allergic reactions.

5. *Misconception:* Fluoride causes blood anomalies.

   Fact: Laboratory tests comparing populations consuming fluoridated and nonfluoridated water reveal no significant differences in the incidence of blood anomalies.

6. *Misconception:* Fluoride causes brittle bones or bone cancer.

   Fact: Numerous studies have found no harmful effects at the concentration recommended for dental health.

7. *Misconception:* Fluoridation equipment is not safe.

   Fact: The development and use of reliable continuous fluoride analyzers in conjunction with modern fluoride-feed systems ensure safe communal water supplies.

with whether fluoridation works as a protection against dental disease.

I think the main reason every community in the United States doesn't have a fluoridated water supply is simply that local authorities don't want to spend the money. They have decided it isn't worth it. They don't know that it helps

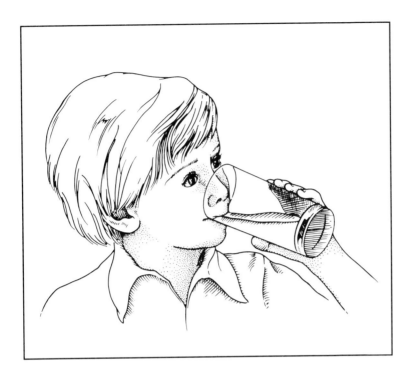

Children who drink fluoridated "city" water have been shown to have 50% to 75% less dental disease. Parents in cities with a fluoridated water supply should therefore encourage their children to drink tap water.

everybody—adults, teenagers, and, most of all, the children in the community.

What Are Fluorides?

Fluorides are a large group of chemical compounds formed when fluorine combines with other elements. Fluorine is never found by itself in nature. Fluorides are found everywhere—in soil, air, and water, as well as in plant and animal life. That's why most foods contain some fluoride. It's estimated that we all consume a baseline level of about 0.3 milligrams of fluoride daily from food and drink.

Minerals are unevenly distributed in the soil of the world, so it follows that the water and foods from one region may contain a high fluoride count, while those of another contain a low count. What we eat and drink will not supply these diet elements in a steady, balanced way, so we sometimes add them to our diets in the proper amounts.

We call fluoride an additive, but that's not really accurate. We are *supplementing* the fluoride in—not introducing it to— the water supply, adjusting the proportions to achieve the optimum balance that will enhance the strength of teeth.

Why the water supply? For one thing, it's the principal natural source of fluorides. As a public health measure, fluoridating water is the one way to reach the most people. We have other ways of adding fluoride to the diet, but they would require every parent and every child to be responsible for the additional fluoride every day. Such a system would never fit into the commitment to prevention—for today and for future generations.

How Does Fluoride Work?

The hardest substances in the body are bones and teeth. When the teeth are forming, the minerals needed are brought to the jaw and deposited in the tooth buds by the bloodstream. When one of these minerals, fluoride, is in adequate supply, it is incorporated into the enamel of the tooth, and the resulting mineral structure is stronger than it would be without the fluoride. As a result, the enamel will be more resistant to attack by the acids that form in the mouth and set the stage for decay.

It's important, then, to get fluoride to the teeth when they are mineralizing. That means from birth, when the primary teeth are forming, right through the development of the adult molars and, in the case of wisdom teeth, even later. Children who drink fluoridated water from infancy through the age of 12 or 13 will have teeth that are stronger than they would otherwise be. They can expect to have half the number of cavities, or even less, than they would have had.

Grown-ups may wonder what, if any, advantage fluoridated water has for them. Plenty! Even if an adult has had minimal fluoride exposure previously, fluoridated water provides a surface benefit. When you drink fluoridated water, or take a fluoride supplement, the fluoride you swallow is later returned to your mouth in the saliva. There, it helps replenish what I like to call your "fluoride reservoir."

The Fluoride Reservoir

Years ago, scientists thought that the fluoride incorporated into teeth at the time they formed was the most important in terms of future resistance to cavities. The theory was that if fluoride was an integral part of the tooth structure, the tooth would be less susceptible to decay for a lifetime. Now we've revised our thinking about that.

Recent research has taught us that a major action of

fluoride takes place not deep inside the tooth, but at its surface, when fluoride comes into contact with saliva and plaque.

Fluoride from all sources is stored in the mouth—on the teeth, in the plaque, in saliva, and in the soft tissues—ready for action. This is your fluoride reservoir.

Normally, there is an ongoing exchange of minerals between the tooth enamel and the saliva. When the tooth takes up as much mineral as it gives up, we have a state of balance or equilibrium.

But when you eat, decay-causing bacteria in your mouth begin to feed, producing acid as a by-product. That acid can upset the balance of mineral exchange, causing the tooth enamel to lose more minerals than it takes up. That net loss, or *demineralization*, is the start of a cavity.

But if the fluoride reservoir is full, it's a different story. The same acid that leads to demineralization first triggers release of fluoride stored in the reservoir. Fluoride becomes available right when it's needed, right where it's needed. And that fluoride not only inhibits demineralization but also promotes *remineralization*, rebuilding and reinforcing tooth enamel so that it is even stronger than it was originally. In effect, fluoride "heals" cavities in the early stages of development. Many parents are surprised that pediatric dentists often suggest using topical fluoride to try to re-mineralize a beginning cavity. Only if that approach doesn't work, then the dentist will suggest filling the cavity.

Recent research has taught us that a major action of fluoride takes place not deep inside the tooth, but at its surface, when fluoride comes into contact with saliva and plaque.

Filling Your Child's Fluoride Reservoir

There are two basic ways to get fluoride: swallow it—as with fluoridated water and fluoride supplements, and apply it topically—as with daily fluoride toothpaste, mouth-rinses, or gel treatments at the dentist's office.

Systemic Fluoride

Fluoride taken internally is systemic—it will be incorporated into the system as building blocks and some of it will return to the mouth in saliva.

There are several ways of getting fluoride into the teeth systemically. When the drinking water in your community naturally contains enough fluoride or has been adjusted to the therapeutic level, the effect is both systemic and topical, and everybody benefits. Where this is not possible — in rural areas, for example — the drinking water in the schools may be fluoridated. For children not exposed to fluoridated water, daily fluoride supplements are available as liquid solutions, in tablet form, and in preparations that combine fluoride with vitamins.

Consult your dentist or physician about whether your child should receive a fluoride supplement at home. If supplemental fluoride is prescribed, they will determine the proper dosage and teach you how to use it.

Liquid fluoride supplements, the type dispensed with a medicine dropper or drip bottle, are often prescribed for infants. If you use a liquid supplement, be sure that the desired dose of fluoride is delivered in a fairly large quantity of solution — 4 milliliters is about right. This helps ensure that you won't overdose the child by accidentally dispensing an extra droplet or two.

When children become old enough to manage chewable tablets, they can switch from the infant preparations. Tablets should be chewed well and swished around in the mouth before swallowing.

Remember to treat fluoride supplements like medicine. Store them out of reach of children and use only as directed.

Fluorosis: When Your Child Gets Too Much Fluoride

Fluorosis, which has no clinical significance in the mouth or the rest of the body, is a cosmetic problem . . .

Fluorosis, which has no clinical significance in the mouth or the rest of the body, is a minor cosmetic problem in which the front surfaces of the permanent teeth develop a white, slightly irregular appearance. The cause is too much fluoride ingested at an early age, while the teeth are forming. Children under the age of 3 often swallow toothpaste because they haven't yet learned to spit it out when they brush. Swallowing toothpaste twice a day for someone under age 3 can lead to a mild fluorosis. To ensure that your child isn't swallowing fluoride toothpaste, be sure to closely supervise toothbrushing at least until your child masters the necessary skills.

The effects of fluorosis range from very mild to severe, although severe cases are extremely rare. Mild fluorosis is literally a surface problem that can be easily and quickly treated in the dental office with a vigorous abrasive cleaning.

Very mild fluorosis cannot be detected by parents or even by dentists, unless they've been trained to recognize it. In fact, mild fluorosis often gives teeth a pleasing bright-white look. Mild fluorosis, then, is somewhat like the old riddle about a tree falling in the forest: if no one is there to hear, does it make a sound? Or, in this case, if neither the child nor the parents can see the "discoloration," is it fluorosis?

Topical Fluoride

There's another way to get fluoride to the teeth. In a topical solution—gel, paste, or liquid—fluoride can be wiped or painted or swished around the surface of the tooth.

When you and your child are in the dentist's office for a periodic checkup and cleaning, the dentist may use a topical fluoride treatment for your child.

The protective benefits of topical fluoride treatments are the key to the dental health of children living in communities with nonfluoridated water. But they are also important to children who do drink fluoridated water. For the average child, they add a little more weight on the child's side of the scale—that is, the chances that he or she will have a cavity in the months after treatment drop a few more points. For the child suffering from serious, extensive cavities, topical treatments can help slow up a runaway situation.

Sometimes I'm faced with such a severe case of cavities that I pull out all the stops and try everything—reviewing cleaning techniques, checking the diet, and recommending a daily rinse with a fluoride solution. Home use of topical fluorides, the same kind I use in my office, may be prescribed until things start looking better.

Bringing Fluoride Into Contact With the Tooth Surface

Topical Fluoride Treatments
These are applied by a dentist following a professional cleaning. Most preparations have a pleasant taste, and the treatment takes only a few minutes.

One method is to fill a tray, molded to fit the teeth, with a solution or gel and place it over the teeth for a few minutes.

Ways to Get Fluoride to Your Child's Teeth

- Encourage your child to drink water. All water contains some fluoride.
- Urge your community to bring the fluoride in its water supply up to a cavity-fighting level.
- If prescribed by your dentist, give your child dietary supplements of fluoride in liquid or tablet form.
- Have your child brush twice daily with a fluoride toothpaste—once after breakfast and again before bedtime.
- Have your child rinse with a fluoride mouthrinse after brushing.
- Take your child to the dentist's office for a regular checkup. The dentist will apply a topical fluoride treatment.

Another way is to apply the fluoride solution with cotton applicators and carry it between the teeth with dental floss. Dentists are studying other methods of applying topical fluoride to teeth, including the use of fluoride-containing chewing gum and fluoridated dental floss.

Fluoride Toothpastes

Even if your water supply is adjusted to the proper level of fluoride and your child is going to the dentist for routine topical fluoride treatments, daily use of a fluoride toothpaste is an excellent way to replenish the fluoride reservoir. Read package labels to choose a brand the American Dental Association's Council on Dental Therapeutics has accepted and approved.

Once again, have your child brush twice a day, after breakfast and before bedtime, and supervise young children to ensure that they don't swallow toothpaste while brushing.

Fluoride Mouthrinses

The fluoride mouthrinses on the market today have been tested on school-age children, some of whom drank fluoridated water and some of whom had only nonfluoridated water available. The results of the tests are impressive. If you decide to add a fluoride mouthrinse to your home fluoride program, be sure to use it as directed and see that your child uses it properly. Some types can be swallowed; most should not be.

A Multiple Approach

I think there's no doubt that a balanced multiple fluoride program will pay off for your child, and with good reason. Under optimum conditions, a tooth comes into the mouth with about 800 ppm of fluoride in the outer layer of enamel. I'm talking about the teeth of a child whose drinking water contains 1 ppm of fluoride and whose teeth did not erupt unusually early, but remained in contact with the fluoride-bearing tissue fluids longer.

Now this figure, 800 ppm, is not the optimum level for fluoride. Tests prove that levels of 1,000 ppm and above are associated with resistance to cavities. Therefore, it is what we do after the teeth come in that can pull this level up. All the ways we use to bring fluoride in contact with the tooth are pushing that figure up the scale.

With all the talk about methods, costs, benefits, and statistics on fluoridation, let's not lose sight of the most interesting thing about fluoride: it works.

How Does Your Family Rate in the Fight Against Decay?

- Do you wipe your baby's teeth and gums after feeding?
- Do you and your older children refill your fluoride reservoirs by gentle brushing twice daily with a fluoride toothpaste?
- Do you floss daily to break up plaque?
- Are your children getting enough fluoride? Check with your dentist.
- Are you snacking too often—more than four or five times a day?
- Has your dentist applied protective sealant to the chewing surfaces of your children's back teeth?

Diet and Dental Health

The last decade has brought about tremendous changes in our thinking about the relation of diet to dental health. As an example, compare the diet advice that dentists—including me—were giving a few years ago to what we're saying today.

Not so long ago, we thought sugar was the bad guy when it came to tooth decay. Avoid sweets, we said, especially sticky ones like caramels.

If you haven't heard the latest thoughts on diet yet, you're in for a big surprise.

You Are What You Eat, But . . .

Except for the beneficial micronutrient fluoride, nutrients in the food you eat probably have little effect on whether cavities form in your mouth. Good nutrition certainly contributes to overall good health but cannot ensure that your children will develop strong, disease-resistant teeth.

False. No amount of milk will prevent tooth decay. It's true that milk is an excellent source of calcium, a mineral necessary to the healthy growth of teeth and bones, and children need milk daily as long as they are growing. As such, milk can be recommended as a nutritious snack. But once the crowns of the teeth are fully formed, calcium intake ceases to have much effect.

While we're on the subject of milk, let's consider chocolate-flavored milk for a moment. Chocolate milk is whole, low-fat, or skim milk to which cocoa or chocolate and sweetener have been added. Like whole milk, the chocolate-flavored variety is an excellent source of protein, calcium, and certain vitamins and minerals. An important factor in considering the nutritional benefits of chocolate milk is that children like it.

Many factors influence whether your children will develop cavities, and diet doesn't matter too much if you pay attention to important steps such as practicing routine hygiene, getting enough fluoride daily, and having your dentist apply a protective sealant to the back teeth.

Food and Tooth Decay

Let's get one thing straight: foods alone don't cause cavities. Many of the foods we eat—including some of the most valuable foods from the standpoint of human nutrition—provide nourishment for oral bacteria. They, in turn, secrete acids that can erode enamel and lead to cavities.

We feed the bacteria in our mouths every time we eat carbohydrates. These come in two types: sugars (simple carbohydrates) and cooked starches (complex carbohydrates) like bread and crackers. Once in the mouth, cooked starches start to be broken down into their component sugars by an enzyme in saliva.

Sweet treats such as cake, cookies, and candy are not measurably worse for your teeth than a hearty meal of spaghetti, bread, fruit salad, and a glass of milk. Refined sugar, *sucrose,* is what people usually think of as "sugar." But dairy products contain a form of sugar called *lactose;* fruits contain another sugar, *fructose;* and cooked starches such as pasta and bread are broken down in the mouth into other sugars, *glucose* and *maltose.*

Recent research shows that some candies are potentially less destructive to the teeth than breads and cookies, and that some fruits (such as apples or bananas), previously considered safe or even protective against cavities, may actually promote decay.

To the bacteria in your mouth, sugar is sugar, no matter what "package" it comes in. So candy isn't "bad" for your teeth, and apples aren't "good" for them, either.

Leisurely Dining, Bacteria Style

Two important factors in our discussion of foods and cavities are how often you eat and how long a particular food stays in the mouth after you eat it.

To survive in a hostile environment such as the mouth, bacteria must take advantage of food when it is available. So, just as your car will start whether the gas tank is full or nearly empty, the bacteria in your mouth become active whether you eat a big meal or a few grapes. And they will remain active—producing acids that can cause cavities—*for at least 30 minutes after you eat.* This is why frequent eating is one factor contributing to tooth decay.

Another is *oral retentiveness,* that is, how long a food remains in the mouth after you eat it. If bacteria could tell you what to eat, they'd probably order foods that stay on and between the teeth for hours after your meal is finished.

What is the stickiest food you can think of? Caramels? Taffy? They feel sticky when you touch them and chewy when you put them into your mouth. But as far as oral retentiveness goes, our tactile perception of stickiness is not accurate. In fact, foods like crackers, muffins, and potato chips—all are cooked starches—stay longer in the mouth than a caramel. The caramel is mostly sugar that dissolves in saliva and clears the mouth fairly quickly. Cooked starches, on the other hand, don't dissolve in saliva and clear the mouth until they have been broken down into their component simple sugars by the salivary enzyme. This process often takes hours, and in the meantime, oral bacteria are making microscopic pigs of themselves and secreting enamel-destroying acids.

Consider what this means if you:
- Eat a cracker that clings to your teeth for more than an hour
- Sip a sugared soft drink throughout the afternoon
- Nurse a sore throat by sucking on sugary lozenges, one after another

Anti-Cavity Foods

At the same time that ideas have changed about what foods promote decay, we've learned more about certain foods that seem to help protect against cavities. Cheese—especially aged cheddar, Monterey Jack, and Swiss—stimulates the flow of saliva, and salivary stimulation may even help repair small breaks in tooth enamel where a cavity has begun to form. Serve cheese as a snack or at the end of a meal.

Is Chocolate Getting a Bad Rap?

Yes. Like most other carbohydrates, chocolate can play a role in the decay process. But it has been unfairly singled out as a major cause of cavities.

What's the point? When research over the last 30 years clearly shows that all foods containing sugars or cooked starches have the potential to promote tooth decay, it's overly simplistic to focus on one food, or 20 foods, as "the worst."

As long as you brush regularly and get sufficient fluoride, there's nothing wrong with snacking sensibly. This can include chocolate—or any other food, for that matter.

In every case, you are subjecting your teeth to prolonged exposure to potentially harmful acids.

The Bottom Line: Diet Is Only Part of the Puzzle

Having read this far, you may wonder whether I'm about to advocate fasting as the unfortunate price you must pay for avoiding cavities. Hardly. I believe that there is a positive side to all this: as long as our children are not constantly snacking, we can stop nagging them about snack selection (at least as far as their teeth are concerned).

Numerous studies from the 1960s showed that the most consistent dietary difference between children with many cavities and those with few or none was not the quantity of carbohydrate foods eaten, but rather how often they were eaten. The 1960s also saw the introduction of fluoride toothpaste; by 1990 the number of people using toothpaste had increased dramatically, and more than 95% of all toothpastes contained fluoride.

Sticky, Stickier, Stickiest

Here is a general guide to the "stickers." It shows how 21 foods studied by dental researchers rank in terms of their apparent ability to cling to the teeth and thereby contribute to the formation of cavities.

Barely sticky: apples, bananas, hot fudge sundaes, milk chocolate bars

Moderately sticky: white bread, caramels, creme-filled sponge cake

Stickier: dried figs, jelly beans, plain doughnuts, raisins

Stickiest: granola bars, oatmeal cookies, potato chips, salted crackers, puffed oat cereal, creme-filled sandwich cookies, peanut butter crackers

With the majority of the population now using fluoride toothpaste, even the issue of frequency of eating has become less significant than it was in the past. As I indicated at the beginning of this chapter, concepts concerning diet and cavities have changed dramatically. Today, there is decreased emphasis on dietary counseling as the most effective strategy to prevent cavities in children. The traditional advice to avoid sticky sweets and between-meal snacks is being relaxed for most cavity-free children who are exposed to fluoride and comprehensive dental care. Many children need snacks daily to help meet their nutritional needs, and parents should choose and offer snack foods accordingly.

Most children can safely snack three or four times a day, in addition to regular meals. This number should be dentally harmless for the child who:

- Brushes thoroughly twice daily with a fluoride toothpaste
- Gets sufficient fluoride from sources such as drinking water, over-the-counter fluoride toothpastes, and topical fluoride treatments applied by the dentist
- Has protective sealant applied to the chewing surfaces of the teeth
- Sees a dentist regularly

True or False?

"Chewing gum helps to clean teeth."

Not exactly. Chewing gum does not clean teeth; only brushing and flossing will clean teeth.

But more and more dentists today recommend chewing sugarless gum after a snack or a meal. Why? Because chewing gum stimulates saliva, and **saliva** *helps wash food particles from the teeth. So, in a roundabout way, gum can have a cleansing effect. Equally important, saliva contains buffers that work to neutralize the acid produced by oral bacteria. Saliva also brings minerals and fluoride to the tooth surface, helping to prevent loss of mineral from the tooth and even to heal early cavities. (For more about saliva, see Chapter 3.)*

A Visit to the Dentist

Choosing a Dentist

The American Academy of Pediatric Dentistry recommends that you take your child to the dentist soon after the first tooth erupts—usually between the ages of 6 months and 1 year. That means you need to find a good dentist for your child, and it's never too early to start your search.

First, ask yourself, what are you looking for in a dentist? Clinical skill and a fine professional reputation are both desirable. But there's another quality that's so obvious it may be overlooked: *find a dentist who likes working with children*. An old saw in dentistry says that there are more dentists who are afraid of children than there are children who are afraid of dentists. Your child's dentist should be patient and considerate, someone who understands the child's point of view and takes the time to help the youngster feel secure in a strange, new setting.

There are a number of ways to find such a dentist, starting with word of mouth (no pun intended). Referrals from satisfied friends or relatives are hard to beat, so ask people you trust whether they would recommend the dentist who treats them or their children. If no one among your acquaintances can recommend a dentist, ask your own family doctor or dentist. Specify that you are looking for a well-qualified dentist who has a special ability for dealing with children.

If you still haven't turned up the name of a likely candidate or two, call the local dental society. Most towns and cities have one. Ask for the names of dentists who like to work with children. You can also look in your local library for the American Dental Association's directory, which lists such specialties as pediatric dentistry. Or you can telephone the nearest accredited hospital and ask the chief of dental service or the attending dentist to recommend several qualified dentists. In general, a personal recommendation is preferable.

Should You Choose a Pediatric Dentist?

While I'm not going to say absolutely that your child ought to have a pediatric dentist, I urge you to consider this option.

Pediatric dentists are the pediatricians of dentistry. They are dedicated to meeting the unique dental health needs of all children, including those with disabilities or special needs. Yet pediatric dentists are no more expensive than general practitioners.

In addition to the standard dental degree, pediatric dentists complete 2 to 3 more years of postgraduate training with emphasis in child psychology and growth and development. To stay current in their specialty, most pediatric dentists belong to the American Academy of Pediatric Dentistry (AAPD), a professional organization dedicated to keeping its membership up to date on the latest techniques of child, infant, and adolescent care. Members often display the AAPD seal in their office or perhaps on their business stationery.

Pediatric dentists are focused on preventive dentistry and can help you and your children understand what causes dental disease and how to prevent it. Their specialized training means they can often detect early signs of developing problems and recommend appropriate corrective action. For example, many orthodontic problems, when caught early, can be prevented without braces or costly, lengthy treatment (see Chapter 8 for more on this).

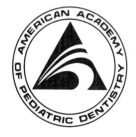

Pediatric dentists who belong to the American Academy of Pediatric Dentistry usually display this seal.

A growing number of pediatric dentists believe so strongly in the preventive approach to dental health that they have designed their offices to de-emphasize the use of drills or other equipment to fill cavities; their emphasis is on helping children grow up cavity free with straight teeth. Other pediatric dentists even self-insure their patients: if a child brushes faithfully twice a day with a fluoride toothpaste and visits the office every 6 months, any cavity that develops will be treated by the dentist at no charge.

While you as a parent should be concerned about the clinical expertise of your child's dentist, your child will probably be far more interested in other aspects of a pediatric dental practice. These dental offices are designed to make children feel at ease. You can expect to find colorful decor, toys and games to occupy restless youngsters, plenty of educational materials, and scaled-down furnishings sized for half-pint patients.

It stands to reason that anyone willing to invest the extra time and money in specialized pediatric dental training must really want to work with children.

Finally, there may be no more persuasive argument in favor of pediatric dentists than this: It stands to reason that anyone willing to invest the extra time and money in specialized pediatric dental training must really want to work with children.

Evaluating a Dentist

Whether you choose a pediatric dentist or general practitioner, take the time to find a dentist before you need one. That way, you can do your homework and make a reasoned, informed choice. You may want to pay a brief call on the dentist before your child's first professional visit. Ask for a tour of the offices and a conference with the dentist. Explain that you are looking for a special kind of dentist and try to get a feel for the doctor's personality, expertise, and approach.

I believe that you can expect the dentist and staff to be familiar with dental disease, the techniques for identifying and removing plaque, the role of nutrition, eating habits, and the optimal use of systemic and topical fluorides. You might expect the dentist to know about the application of sealants. And you'd expect skillful and painless repair, if needed, with the latest dental techniques and equipment.

*A dentist should not be
concerned only with repair
work, and neither should you.*

Try to determine whether the dentist is concerned about the growth and development of your child by noting whether he or she seems more concerned with filling teeth (is cavity-oriented) than with *preventing* cavities in the first place. A dentist should not be concerned only with repair work, and neither should you. Reading this book should give you not only a broad knowledge of your child's teeth, but also the clues you'll need to know whether a dentist's orientation is toward the *whole* child.

Remember, the most valuable commodities a dentist has to sell are time, skill, and a genuine interest in your child—not little bits of silver filling or x-ray film.

How to Help Your Child Have a Pleasant Experience at the Dentist's Office

Making haste slowly is truly the best policy when a child visits the dentist. If the experience is to be a pleasant one, it's important that the dentist and parents try to avoid alarming the child. In my own practice, I've always tried to accommodate the young patient as much as possible.

An Infant's First Dental Visit

Your child's first visit to the dentist will probably be made between the ages of 6 months and 1 year—when the first tooth comes in. Obviously, a child of that age requires special handling.

When a parent brings in such a youngster, I generally do the oral exam with the child lying or sitting in the parent's lap. Or, if the baby is more comfortable upright looking over the parent's shoulder, I step behind the dental chair and do the exam from that vantage point.

To avoid startling the baby, all my movements will be slow and gentle. And the exam itself will be as brief as possible, using no tools or instruments in the patient's mouth. I check the baby's facial and oral development, the gum pads, and the soft tissues to verify that everything looks healthy and normal and to assess any problems such as tongue tie.

The balance of this first visit is informational. I explain how to clean the baby's mouth and have the parent do the job while I observe and check technique. We also discuss the importance of fluoride and how to ensure that the baby gets the amount needed. If I do my job well, all three of us—doctor, patient, and parent—will have a pleasant and worthwhile first visit.

Older Children Need Special Handling, Too

It's equally important to maintain an atmosphere of security and comfort during subsequent dental visits. For example, when a toddler visits my office, I ask if he/she would like to climb into the chair; to lift the child suddenly and without approval could cause a terrific loss of dignity. I sit, so we can talk eye to eye, and I speak in a low, calm voice to avoid producing any more excitement than is already present in the situation.

I don't want to penetrate the child's personal space too abruptly, so I reach out—at arm's length—and take the child's hand. Counting the child's fingers (counting is a calm, prosaic procedure), I slowly draw closer to the chair. I think of the process as tell/show/do: I tell the child everything I am going to do, show how I am going to do it, and then do exactly what I have said.

I invite my young patient to look around, take a drink of water, hold a small hand mirror while we look at his/her mouth and count the teeth together. Watching what is going on is not only absorbing; it keeps the child from imagining all sorts of things that are not going on. If I am going to accomplish the dental exam and any treatment required, I must stay attuned to the child's responses and proceed at his or her pace.

My objective is always to provide quality dental care while respecting my young patient's needs and feelings.

Getting Ready for a Visit

I know you feel you should prepare your child for a visit to the dentist, but the less prepping you do, the better. Don't promise that the dentist will do nothing more than look at the child's teeth. If the office is new to you, don't even try to describe what it will look like or what the office procedure will be.

Much to the surprise of most parents and many dentists, children tolerate local anesthesia quite well.

Don't try to discuss the dentist's equipment. You might use words that could inadvertently alarm the child. In my office, for instance, a pick or an explorer is a "tooth-feeler"; a drill is a "tooth-cleaner"; fluoride solution is called a "tooth-shiner"; and words and phrases such as "hurt," "shot," "Novocaine," "injections," and "pinch you with a needle" are not in my vocabulary. If I must do some work that will "bother" (not "hurt") the child, then I "put the tooth to sleep." Much to the surprise of most parents and many dentists, children tolerate local anesthesia quite well.

Letting children listen to the words the dentist uses, form their own impressions, and experience their own sensations makes them better able to deal with it all.

Too often, children who are brought to the dentist expect something entirely different from the experience that awaits them. If, for example, you tell your child, "This is not going to hurt," you have planted the notion of pain in your child's head. And with today's modern techniques, including topical anesthesia, the dentist isn't likely to hurt your child. Should treatment involve some discomfort, dentist and patient can get through it together if confidence has been built from the very first visit.

Try to Control Your Own Anxieties

It's difficult for parents who themselves have had bad dental experiences to bring their children to the dentist without keying them in to their own fears. Children have sensitive antennae.

Here's an old parent trick. You're taking your child to the dentist, and your own anxiety leads you to promise to buy the child a toy, a comic book, or an ice-cream soda when the visit is over. The child knows something's up. Why would you be offering a treat in the middle of the afternoon? It's not even a special day. Or is it?

The parent's hand tightens and voice gets a little higher. The parent grimaces, face muscles taut. The child takes it all in.

I know it's difficult to hide your feelings. The best advice I have for you as a parent is that you try to believe that going to the dentist can be a nonthreatening, non-fear-provoking experience. It can even be a good experience. Try to forget your own prejudices and keep an open mind. Let your child come to the office without carrying the burden of your apprehension.

Should You Accompany Your Child Into the Treatment Room?

The answer to this question depends on three people: parent, child, and dentist.

Some parents do not have the ability to hand their children over to someone else's care, regardless of the confidence they may feel in the other person. They feel they have to protect, intervene, interpret.

Children may be comfortable in the unfamiliar environment of the dentist's office if they can see a familiar face. On the other hand, children of even 3 or 4 may want Mommy or Daddy there because they believe it will protect them or they know they can manipulate their parents by fussing or crying; the dentist is an unknown entity. It's not inconceivable that your 4-year-old is taking the occasion to embarrass you, the parent who brought him/her here.

If you panic at hearing your child cry in the office, just stop and listen for a moment. Is this plain, everyday crying? Is it different from the child's crying when he/she wants to go skating or to have bedtime put off a little longer? Is it that special crying within your child's arsenal—the "atom bomb"? If it's familiar, treat it as you would under ordinary circumstances.

As for the dentist, some are not comfortable with an audience but prefer working and relating one-to-one with the child. Other dentists are more extroverted and are not uncomfortable working in front of the parent and an assistant. Personality comes into it. Let the dentist make the decision.

If you are asked to stay in the treatment room, it's usually best if you will stay out of your child's vision. It only takes one fleeting wince or concerned look on your face to inadvertently alarm your observant child. And as much as you want to reassure your child, I think it's best if you don't talk. Don't say, "This will be over in a minute," or "Wait till I tell Daddy how you behaved in the dentist's office." Please resist the temptation to applaud your child's good behavior or to reprimand your child when he/she doesn't cooperate.

Personally, I like the parent in the treatment room if he or she is a silent observer and sits behind the child so as not to provide facial or body cues. Sometimes it's most comforting for a preschooler to hold a parent's hand, and an infant or a very young child is often most at ease while sitting in the parent's lap.

Sometimes it's most comforting for a preschooler to hold a parent's hand, and an infant or a very young child is often most at ease while sitting in the parent's lap.

I've gone into all this to explain how certain methods work for me. I call them my "superstitions," the procedures and techniques that I find most effective. Your dentist may be equally comfortable and successful working in different ways from those I describe.

A Visit to the Dentist Differs From a Visit to the Pediatrician

Going to the dentist is not the same as going to a pediatrician, and parents shouldn't expect one experience to be comparable to the other. The dentist faces different problems. First, the child's cooperation is essential. To do a proper cleaning, an accurate x-ray, or a good restoration, the dentist needs the child's attention for as long as 15 to 20 minutes at a time. The pediatrician, who puts a child on a scale, looks in the child's throat, and listens to the child's chest, needs a shorter period of cooperation.

Parents often help the pediatrician by holding or supporting the child. Because they don't perceive the visit to the pediatrician as a threatening situation, they don't transmit tension to the child.

Another difference: Often the child has to come to the dentist for a repeated number of visits, so the dentist must sustain the relationship from one visit to the next. Pediatric visits are generally separated by longer periods of time once the child is past infancy.

What do you do if you bring two children to the office — say, one 3-year-old and one 5-year-old? Do you put big brother in the chair and let his younger sister watch?

Although it may surprise you — and perhaps your dentist — I advise letting the younger child go first. Why? Because if little sister goes first and behaves well, the older child will feel that he must do as well. Also, the younger one has no way of interpreting what's being done to her big brother, so watching won't prepare her for her own experience. And she may resent always being the second banana.

I wouldn't worry about the effects of your child's crying on other children, who generally recognize crying for what it is: frustration, anger, or a need for attention.

If you feel you must prepare the child for a visit to the dentist, follow the rule that applies to sex and politics: tell the child no more than he or she is ready to hear. I myself would say something like this: "We're going to the dentist this afternoon. The dentist is going to look at your teeth. When we get there you can sit in a special chair. The dentist will look in your mouth, count your teeth, and tell you a little bit about how to take care of them."

Unfortunately, some children never see a dentist until there's an emergency. The family has waited until a cavity has developed or a toothache has come along. In that case, you could say: "A dentist is someone who takes care of your teeth when they hurt and fixes them so they can get better. That's why we're going to the dentist."

As with any new subject, you should answer only the questions your child asks, giving information on the appropriate level, and no more than the child wants to know at that time. And when you don't know something, it's better to admit it rather than make up an answer.

Unfortunately, some children never see a dentist until there's an emergency.

Safety in the Dental Office

I suspect that more and more people these days wonder whether a visit to the dentist may result in exposure to some infectious disease. In fact, dental health professionals share those concerns.

The nature of our work means that we risk daily contact with organisms that cause everything from the common cold and flu to hepatitis and even AIDS. The potential is there for the dentist or hygienist to catch something from—or spread it to—a patient. I point this out not to frighten you, but to reassure you that the dental profession is well aware of the potential.

Organizations like the American Dental Association and the Centers for Disease Control have thought through the risks and devised stringent infection-control recommendations that most dental offices follow scrupulously. You'll notice that dentists and assistants these days wear surgical gloves, face masks, and even goggles during dental procedures. That's probably the most obvious sign that we're being more careful than ever. But behind the scenes, we're taking other precautions to protect our patients and ourselves. We disinfect surfaces in the treatment room between patients, we sterilize instruments after every use, and we routinely test our sterilization equipment to make sure it's working properly. Also, our staff members have all their inoculations up to date and receive semi-annual health checkups.

If you have any reservations about the issue of infection control, don't hesitate to ask your dentist or an assistant about their procedures. They will be happy to answer your questions.

How Often Should You Visit the Dentist?

In general, dental visits should take place every 6 months, but that can vary. Some children are more susceptible to decay than others; some have better dental hygiene habits than others; some eat more often than others. Regular and frequent visits give the dentist an opportunity to discover problems early, which lowers the chances of the child's suffering pain, serious complications, and loss of teeth. Routine visits pay for themselves in the long run by helping to head off costly problems.

X-ray Examinations

The x-ray is a valuable diagnostic tool for the dentist. Decay can proceed so rapidly in children that it is important to detect a cavity as soon as possible. Cavities still too small to be seen by the naked eye will show up on an x-ray. And decay spots between the teeth, where a mirror and explorer can't reach, can be located by x-ray.

Extra teeth, missing teeth—any anomaly in the permanent teeth, which are still buried in the jaw—can be seen on x-rays. This information is needed if the dentist must decide whether to retain or remove teeth.

Parents, dentists, and physicians are justifiably concerned about the proliferating and extensive use of x-rays. There is

X-rays allow the dentist to visualize the state of development of the permanent teeth and to determine whether there are any cavities between the teeth. Notice the developing permanent teeth beneath the gums of this normal 2½-year-old (left) and 6½-year-old (right).

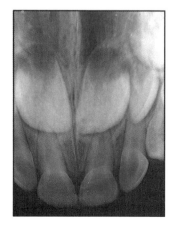
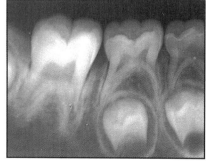

incontrovertible evidence that people who receive excessive x-ray therapy as children may develop problems. Excessive use of x-rays should be avoided whenever possible.

Today's machines are safe and easily operated. When I finished dental school, an x-ray took 1 or 1.5 seconds of exposure time. Today, new, shielded equipment takes the same x-rays in tenths of a second; 15 or 20 pictures can be taken in the time it took for one of the old-style exposures. The amount of radiation from once-a-year x-rays is less than the child would get from natural sources during a day at the beach. And in my office a child who has good 6-month reports doesn't get an x-ray at every visit.

Special x-ray machines can take a single panoramic picture of the jaws. The child sits still, and the film, in a flexible cassette, is placed on a rotating drum. It shifts around and takes a full view of all primary and permanent teeth. This, with a few cavity-checking pictures, should be enough for the dentist's initial diagnostic needs.

Anesthesia

There may be times when a young child—a preschooler, perhaps—has to have extensive dentistry done (maybe oral surgery) and the dentist may suggest general anesthesia.

General Anesthesia

I think all parents should be aware that general anesthesia used on young children entails a risk. Children who lose consciousness under general anesthesia lose their protective reflexes. Because of their small body size, they carry a smaller amount of oxygen in their lungs than adults. For young children there are risks that adults—or even 9- or 10-year-olds—do not face.

I believe this is a case when it's advisable to have the anesthesia done by a specialist who works just with children. The pediatric dentist's training in psychology and treatment of young children may enable him or her to do the work under local anesthesia. Tragedies do occur under general anesthesia. If I must use it—and there are times when I have no choice but to do so—I always advise that the procedure be performed in a hospital, where the anes-

. . . all parents should be aware that general anesthesia used on young children entails a risk.

thesia is administered by an anesthesiologist—a physician who specializes in this field. This reduces risk. If I can, I arrange to have a pediatric anesthesiologist assist me. The specialist concentrates on anesthetic management and I am free to concentrate on my work.

Local Anesthesia

Most adults have grown up with a fear of needles and injections. But today it is entirely possible to give a child an injection that involves nothing more than the slightest pulling sensation.

Dentists are trained to administer local anesthetics and can do so with skill. The psychological preparation of dentist and child is important.

All About Orthodontics

What I am going to say here will sound controversial to some orthodontists and confusing to some parents, but when you think about it, it's logical.

When Is Orthodontics Needed?

Orthodontic Treatment to Improve Appearance

By and large, most people seek orthodontic treatment because their teeth don't look good. That is, appearance is the primary motivation for orthodontic therapy.

It is a strong, valid reason. We live in a world where a bright smile and straight, even teeth contribute to social and professional success. The lack of such a smile leads to self-consciousness and misery. Most parents do not want their child to be handicapped by an unattractive appearance.

Some people think that teeth that are straight, well-spaced, well-aligned, and lacking an overbite are healthy teeth. Not necessarily. They're just pretty. For the most part, crooked teeth are not inherently unhealthy teeth. A couple of rotated teeth in the front of the mouth might create a cleaning problem, but in general, spaces, leaning teeth, and crookedness are neither dangerous nor unhealthy.

Medical Reasons for Orthodontic Therapy

There are some rare instances where orthodontics becomes medically necessary. Examples of these are inherited disorders, such as infantile osteomyelitis (a chronic infection of the bones); accidents and injuries; and a form of ankylosis (abnormal bone fusion) in which partially unerupted permanent teeth become fused with the jawbone and stop short of arriving fully in the mouth. But these are rare conditions.

Should Your Child Have Orthodontics?

If I were a parent contemplating orthodontics for my child, I would first find out whether the child is dissatisfied with the appearance of his or her teeth. If both the parents and the child feel strongly that the appearance is unsightly, then it is reasonable to choose treatment.

Occlusion

There is no absolute standard for the way teeth fit or look. Teeth have as much individuality as people do.

Occlusion—the way the teeth fit together when the jaw is closed—is different in each person. Occlusion also changes throughout a person's life—as primary teeth are shed, adult teeth arrive, growth patterns change, and wear and habit accomplish their effects.

When occlusion is good, both sides of the jaw and face are matching, or symmetrical. You probably would not notice a slight sideward swing of the lower jaw, a sign of malocclusion, which is discussed below. If you want to look at your child's teeth in occlusion, instead of asking to "open up," ask your child to show you his or her mouth with the lips open and teeth closed.

There is no absolute standard for the way teeth fit or look. Teeth have as much individuality as people do.

Notice that the front teeth project ahead of their matching bottom teeth. That's called *overjet*. The top teeth also extend down, covering their matching lower teeth to some degree. That is called *overbite*. These are normal conditions.

It's quite a surprise to parents when the small, neat, white primary teeth are lost and the enormous, ivory permanent teeth erupt. After all, these are fully grown adult teeth coming into a jaw and face that still belong to a child. Especially during the months of mixed dentition, when your child shows a mixture of primary teeth, adult teeth, and gaps, you may wonder whether there's something wrong. I assure you, this is a perfectly natural and temporary stage of the child's dental development.

Malocclusion

Any deviation from the normal way in which the teeth of the upper jaw meet and fit with the teeth of the lower jaw is called *malocclusion*.

Please don't try to diagnose malocclusion on your own. If you think your child may have a problem, seek the advice of a dental professional who is specially trained and experienced in dental and facial development.

Preventive Orthodontics

In recent years, the dental profession has revised some of its ideas about orthodontics. We now know that many

Malocclusion Can Cause Problems

- When teeth don't meet properly, they may not be able to perform normal cutting and grinding functions. This sometimes causes people to avoid foods needed in a balanced and varied diet simply because they are just too difficult to eat.
- If there is displacement of the lower jaw in relation to the upper jaw, resulting problems may include lack of symmetry, pressure on the front portion of the ear, or pain in the jaw hinge (temporomandibular joint).
- An individual who is unhappy about his or her appearance may suffer lack of confidence and poor self-image.

. . . much expensive and lengthy orthodontic treatment can be avoided by taking preventive steps when the child is as young as 4 or 5.

malocclusions can be recognized and treated much earlier than was once common practice. In fact, many pediatric dentists now believe that much expensive and lengthy orthodontic treatment in the teen years can be avoided by taking preventive steps when the child is as young as 4 or 5.

The general dental practitioner or the pediatric dentist who has been seeing your child in the early years can and does practice preventive orthodontics. How? By trying to prevent the premature loss of primary teeth due to decay or accident; by saving room for adult teeth when primary teeth are prematurely lost; and by repairing primary teeth, when necessary, accurately and carefully to maintain the tooth's shape and function. These things are effective in an orthodontic dimension, too.

Space Maintainers

Suppose a primary tooth is lost before it should be, perhaps knocked out in a fall. Your dentist may recommend the use of a temporary space maintainer, a device that will hold the space open until the permanent tooth is ready to grow into its proper position. A similar device sometimes is used to regain space already lost.

Maintaining the space, however, is not always necessary. In the front of the mouth, space seems to stabilize. If a space maintainer is needed anywhere, it is usually in the back of the mouth. It is important to keep the appropriate relationships in the back teeth, but even here, a space maintainer is not always needed.

What can happen if the space is not saved when it should be? The teeth on each side may begin to tip over into the space. The matching tooth in the opposite jaw, meeting no resistance, will grow longer. Drifting teeth cause the stresses of chewing to be distributed unevenly, which is not good for the supporting bones and gums. It's a situation that may call, in a few years, for a full set of braces.

Keeping an Eye on Your Child's Mouth

It's just as important to keep watch for teeth that are retained too long. When primary teeth stay around after they should be gone, they leave the incoming permanent teeth with nowhere to go but sideways. If you become familiar with your child's mouth and have made a practice of counting your child's teeth, you will become aware if a baby tooth has been around longer than it should be.

Watching Out for Bad Mouth Habits

When a tooth comes into the mouth, it doesn't know where it's going. It follows the path of least resistance and responds to the environment in which it finds itself. Among the most important environmental factors determining the position of the permanent teeth are muscular habits, such as thrusting the tongue against the upper teeth with each swallow, biting the lower lip, and thumb sucking. After the child is 6, when the permanent teeth begin to come in, these habits often lead to problems.

If your child has a bad habit, here are two important questions to ask your child's dentist: "Is my child's habit likely to cause malocclusion?" "Is there anything we can do now to prevent a problem later?"

The preventive dentistry that deals with troublesome habits is called "interceptive orthodontics." If a developing orthodontic problem can be intercepted, many malocclusions can be prevented entirely, or treatment can be greatly reduced. It may be as simple as performing an exercise with a wooden tongue depressor to control an incipient crossbite in an erupting incisor.

Your child's dentist can advise you if and when you need to consult an orthodontist.

Exercises to Prevent Orthodontic Problems

Many orthodontic problems occur because of imbalances of the muscles in and around the mouth. The teeth find their place in the dental arch because of the forces that work on them, that is, the tongue, the lips, and the cheeks as they move during chewing and swallowing.

A dentist trained in growth and development can detect imbalances and may be able to give your child exercises to strengthen muscles, thereby avoiding use of orthodontic appliances to reposition teeth.

Blowing a ping-pong ball on a string, for instance, develops the lip muscles, while playing a wind instrument such as a bugle or trombone develops both the lips and cheeks. One of the most common muscular habits—pushing the tongue forward during swallowing—can often be remedied by teaching the child to look in a mirror and swallow without wrinkling the muscles of the chin.

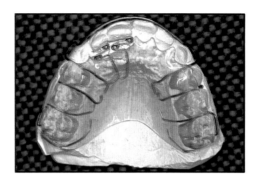

The early use of simple appliances such as this can sometimes eliminate the need for costly and extensive orthodontic therapy.

How Orthodontics Works

Attaining normal occlusion is the job of the pediatric dentist. Regaining normal occlusion is the job of the orthodontist. Orthodontics includes both preventive and corrective measures, and an orthodontist has had postgraduate work in this specialty.

The physiologic basis for orthodontics is the fact that bone is not as hard and unyielding as we generally think. Bone is flexible and malleable. The dentist, by applying long-term gentle pressure with various appliances and through exercises, can gradually bring teeth back into occlusion. Bone yields to the pressure in front of the tooth, and new bone forms and hardens behind it.

The basic appliances and materials used in orthodontics have not changed much over the years: springs, wires, rubber bands, and braces with plastic, metal, or ceramic brackets, some attached and some removable. But there are more options available today than there were 20 years ago. The old "metal mouth" look can be avoided, for instance, by using white or clear brackets that are nearly invisible. Not that braces are much of a stigma anymore. Wearing them seems to be "in"; it's a sign of self-esteem, and children are more nonchalant about orthodontia than they used to be. Besides, much of the orthodontic work being done today is completed before the self-conscious teen years.

. . . much of the orthodontic work being done today is completed before the self-conscious teen years.

Choosing an Orthodontist

Choosing an orthodontist is a big step. Like plastic surgery, it's done only once, and the esthetic result is one that the child will have to live with throughout life. In financial

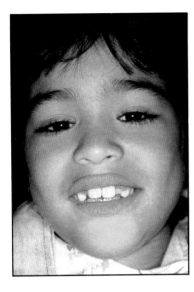
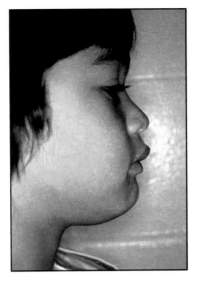
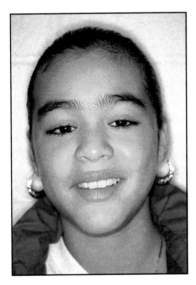
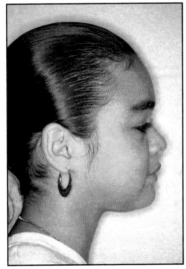

This young lady was 9 years of age when she began orthodontic treatment (top). She was 11½ when it was completed.

terms, it's like buying a car: it's expensive.

Most orthodontists will take a series of x-rays and make study casts of the child's mouth in preparing a treatment plan. If you want another opinion as to the mode of treatment or cost or anything else, don't be embarrassed to ask the orthodontist to send your child's records to another orthodontist for a second opinion. It's done all the time. I myself am quite pleased to send my records to someone else for evaluation. To me, such a request means that the parents are going to be actively involved in the treatment decisions. And that leads to better treatment for the child.

... it is customary and proper for one dentist to send casts and x-rays to another dentist at your request.

Some cautions, however:
- Don't be upset if a second orthodontist recommends a different course of treatment. There are many different appliances and ways of achieving a healthy, esthetic result. In asking for another opinion, you always run the risk of confusing yourself. If this should happen, keep asking questions until you and your child feel comfortable choosing which advice to follow. Fortunately, when it comes to orthodontics, there are no emergencies.
- Don't expect the orthodontist to give the study casts and x-rays to you. Surprisingly, the law says that they belong to the dentist. However, it is customary and proper for one dentist to send casts and x-rays to another dentist at your request.

How Long Will It Take?

An orthodontist usually won't be able to tell you exactly how long treatment will take. Each patient's situation is unique.

If too much pressure is applied when a tooth is moved through bone with an appliance, the root of the tooth may be resorbed. In other words, too much pressure from the appliance can loosen a tooth—even extract it! The dentist must apply just the right amount of pressure on the tooth to move it without letting the root be lost. That's why you may have to expect 2½ or perhaps even 3½ years for orthodontics to be completed. You just can't rush it.

There are other factors that can influence the length of the treatment. Children grow at different rates, and no one can predict how much growth will occur during any course of treatment. Also, the child's cooperation with the treatment is important. Without it, treatment can take many extra months.

How Much Will It Cost?

Many parents wonder why orthodontics is so expensive. Tooth movement takes a great deal of planning by the dentist before the braces go on. And a great deal of time must be spent in making adjustments. It is not uncommon for a child to visit the orthodontist for half an hour every 2 weeks. Over a period of 3 years, this really adds up.

Most orthodontists will evaluate your child's case and give you an estimate of the time and cost involved for treatment. Corrective orthodontia is often covered by dental insurance. If you are not covered, however, most doctors will work out an installment payment plan so you can spread the cost of the treatment over time.

How Much Will It Hurt?

Orthodontics should be painless. If your child's teeth feel sore for several days after an adjustment, tell the orthodontist; the braces may be too tight.

If a protruding spot on a wire or band is irritating or cutting the tissue of the mouth, you or your child can cover the protrusion with a bit of soft paraffin or sugarless chewing gum. That will make things more comfortable until the orthodontist can correct the problem.

Removable or Fixed Appliances?

The question of whether removable or fixed appliances should be used has to be decided by the dentist. Removable appliances (sometimes called "retainers") are mostly used for minor or short-term corrections (6 months to a year).

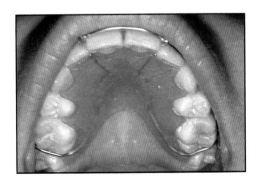

Although they look complicated and appear uncomfortable to wear, removable appliances (sometimes referred to as "retainers") are well tolerated by children.

For major, long-term work, the fixed appliance gives the dentist more control because success doesn't depend on the child's remembering to wear it. No matter how careful everyone promises to be, removable appliances are always getting lost in the cafeteria or at the bottom of a swimming pool, or getting sat on in someone's back pocket. The need for constant repair or replacement is not only expensive; it's an irritation for the child, parents, and dentist.

Oral Hygiene During Orthodontics

Tooth movement is dangerous for somebody who has a high caries history. Dental caries, as noted before, is a multifactorial disease. Bands and braces may be just that extra factor that weights the decay balance on the negative side.

Children wearing tooth-moving appliances have to make an extra effort to keep their mouths clean. It is heartbreaking to have a child enter orthodontic treatment with no cavities, and then find, when the bands and braces are removed, nice straight teeth full of decay. You might consider adding a water-irrigating device to your tooth-cleaning equipment while your child undergoes treatment. Daily use of a fluoride mouthrinse is also a good idea.

Preventing Dental Problems: Past, Present, Future

Background of the Preventive Dentistry Movement

In the late 1960s and early 1970s, there was a great and enthusiastic movement throughout the United States among dentists and in schools and health education programs for a concept called "preventive dentistry." The control of dental disease seemed within our grasp, and it was an exciting time.

What triggered this movement was exact information from laboratories in scientific fields as diverse as physical chemistry, oral microbiology, and nutritional biochemistry. For the first time, we knew exactly what happens in the formation of cavities. We thought we had known for a long time, but now we had clinical proof.

Many of us were encouraged to think that if we could eliminate the dental plaque that leads to cavities, we could eliminate dental disease for all time! Dentists, parents, and teachers all mounted an attack on plaque. The focus of this effort was the identification of plaque by the use of disclosing

True or False?

"Losing teeth is just part of getting old—like gray hair and wrinkles. Sooner or later, everybody wears dentures."

Nonsense. Teeth were designed to last as long as you do. With proper care, at home and at the dentist's office, you and your child can keep your teeth for a lifetime—a long one.

solutions, and then its removal by brushing and flossing.

The problem is that, although it's theoretically possible to prevent the formation of cavities and most gum problems with a program of vigorous brushing and flossing twice a day, it's difficult to make people stick to such a program. For too many people, children and adults alike, the personal effort just doesn't become a routine, like combing your hair or tying your shoelaces. In one study involving dental students, who certainly knew all about plaque and who had access to any specialized dental instruments they wanted to help remove it, most of them failed to completely remove plaque from their own teeth.

The plaque control challenge is not so different from two other health concerns. People know that neither cigarettes nor high-fat diets are good for them. But how many make the effort to change? If doctors can't get people to stop smoking, if they can't get them to eat wisely and exercise, how are they going to motivate them to brush and floss regularly? Just telling people what is good for them is not enough.

Many people, including me, lost confidence in the preventive dentistry movement's "plaque attack" as the means to end cavities in the general population. In theory, it's possible; in practice, it didn't work.

I have not the slightest doubt that I can take a highly motivated child with a highly motivated parent and start them on a program of tooth care that results in immaculate teeth for a period of time. But the question arises: Will they still be so careful 2, 3, or 6 months from now?

The answer is no.

The commitment just doesn't hold up. Yes, there are dentists who can make it work. Dentists can spend all their time constantly urging and supervising their patients in the practice of preventive dentistry. An unusual relationship like that might work, but it entails such dependency and such involvement between dentist and patient that it is impractical and unrealistic. I don't believe patients should become wedded to a dental office in this way.

My father was a dentist, a devoted practitioner of preventive dentistry. He believed that it's the way to prevent dental disease. I don't. I believe our best hope is to focus on a few things that we know work well. In the past, we talked about many things, hoping that parents would do some of them. Today, we've distilled our recommendations down to five key points. These are the things we know are most effective in preventing dental disease.

The Five Key Tools for Preventing Dental Problems

1. **Brush thoroughly twice daily** with a fluoride toothpaste.

2. **Drink fluoridated water** or, on the advice of your dentist or physician, use fluoride supplements. There is no question in my mind or anybody else's that if one child grows up in a neighborhood with a fluoridated water supply, and another has access only to nonfluoridated water, by the time the children are in high school, the one without fluoridated water will have about 50% more cavities than the other. That's a persuasive statistic.

3. **Have sealants applied to the back teeth** soon after they erupt. Eight out of 10 cavities in children under age 12 form on the chewing surfaces of the back teeth—precisely the territory that sealants were developed to protect.

4. **Snack in moderation.** Remember, oral bacteria aren't too fussy about *what* you eat; they'll eat it, too. And every time they eat, they produce acid. Limit between-meal snacks to no more than 3 or 4 daily and you'll minimize the number of times your teeth are exposed to acid attack.

5. **Visit the dentist regularly** (twice a year). A periodic professional cleaning and consultation will help ensure your child's optimum dental health.

This defensive dental program can work for your family and make your children members of a cavity-free generation.

The Numbers Game

I know that statistics are dull, and I've tried to avoid them. But statistics have a message, so let's take a look at these:

- A 1987 survey of 40,000 US children between the ages of 5 and 17 found that half had no cavities, and that tooth decay had declined 36% in the 7 years since the last such survey.
- Seven out of 10 children under age 5 today have no cavities. Of those who do, most got them before age 3.
- Ninety percent of pediatric dentists' children under age 12 have no cavities, compared with 50% in the general population of children under 12.

In just a few decades, we've made tremendous progress in the battle against tooth decay. There is, I believe, no reason that we cannot go the distance and completely conquer the problem. It won't be long before we'll be crowing that 85% of all children under age 12 are cavity-free. And one day, maybe, a cavity will be an extraordinary occurrence.

Dentistry of the Future

Research on several fronts has turned up new technologies that are changing dentistry. Not too long ago, for example, we saw the development of new restorative materials that gave us new treatment options. With these new tooth-colored materials, we can often repair a tooth that might otherwise have been a candidate for a cap. We can rebuild a broken corner of an incisor or close up a wide gap between teeth. Teeth that are gray or have an uneven color or texture can be made white, smooth, and shiny in just a few minutes.

Early interceptive techniques to prevent crooked teeth and reduce the need for corrective orthodontia have also become commonplace. One such approach encourages instruction in certain musical instruments—sousaphones and trumpets, for example—to prevent malocclusion. Exercises with ping-pong balls and other devices have also proved successful (see Chapter 8).

I concluded my 1977 book with a series of 19 dental miracles that were at that time in the research and development stages. Today, roughly two thirds of those have moved out of the science laboratory and are being used increasingly around the country. Among them: plaque-removing toothpastes and rinses, chemicals that dissolve tooth decay without drilling, ultrasonic drills and dental cleaning devices, and colorless orthodontic appliances.

So, I've gone back to my crystal ball to give you a peek at some of the future advancements that may be in widespread use by the time I write my next book!

More Upcoming Miracles

- A pleasant-tasting fluoride toothpaste designed for infants that will inhibit plaque formation.

- An effective, once-a-day fluoride toothpaste.

- Easy-to-use sealants that can be applied to children's teeth in the classroom or at home.

- A timed-release fluoride "button" that can be affixed to a tooth to provide months of protection.

- A simple saliva test that will reveal instantly whether a child is likely to get a cavity.

- A safe and effective use-at-home bleach to remove plaque and brighten teeth.

- Nearly invisible mouth guards for contact sports.

- Painless electrical local anesthesia for dental procedures, powered by a flashlight battery.

- Plaque-removing chewing gums to help prevent cavities.

- New diagnostic techniques, such as fiberoptics, as an alternative to dental x-rays.

- Tooth-colored filling materials that contain ingredients to prevent further decay.

- "Dental first-aid kits" available at gyms, playgrounds, and sports arenas, so that if someone has a tooth knocked out it can be safely transported to a dentist for possible reimplantation.

- Sealants to cover and protect the entire tooth.

- Lasers, designed to be used instead of dental drills, that can vaporize enamel painlessly, without the need for anesthesia.

- Toothpastes that keep your breath fresh all day.

Conclusion

If you have read this book through, you now know about as much as any parent needs to know to rear a dentally healthy child.

But I want to add one caution: if, despite all the best efforts of you and your child, the youngster gets a cavity after all, keep your perspective. Please don't try to fix blame: it's not your fault or your child's fault. Cavities are an unfortunate but natural risk of having teeth. And with today's materials and techniques, your dentist can repair a cavity easily, painlessly, and often invisibly.

The information in this book is the most current that we have on how to prevent dental problems. Use it and you will vastly improve your child's chances of growing up cavity free.

Index

A

Accidents, 56, 58–59, 62
Adolescents. *See* Teenagers.
Alveolar bone. *See* Jawbone.
American Academy of Pediatric Dentistry, 99, 115, 116
American Academy of Pediatrics, 99
American Association for Dental Research, 99
American Cancer Society, 99
American Dental Association, 40, 91, 99, 125
American Institute of Nutrition, 99
American Medical Association, 99
American Osteopathic Association, 99
Anesthesia
  general, 125
  local, 126
Ankylosis, 128
Antibiotics, 12, 85

B

Baby-bottle tooth decay, 15–17

Baby teeth. *See* Primary teeth.
Bacteria, oral, 10, 78–79, 110–111
  foods and, 78, 110–111
  plaque and, 82–85
  tooth decay and, 82–84, 110–111
Bad breath, 41, 64
Biting, 20–21
Bottle vs breast feeding, 14, 15, 16
Braces, 33
Breast vs bottle feeding, 14–16
Bruxism. *See* Tooth grinding.
Bulimia, 66

C

Calcium, 6, 71
Canines, 30
Caries. *See* Cavities.
Cavities, 10, 81, 94, 96, 107
  carbohydrates, 83, 110
  full-term babies and, 8
  premature babies and, 8
Cementum, 74

Cerebral palsy,　23
Cheek biting,　45, 46
Chewing,　5, 20–21
Chewing gum,　78, 106, 113
Childhood illness
　prevention,　11
　record of,　12
Children
　anesthesia for,　125–126
　dental care,　67, 70, 115–126
　dental hygiene,　38–40, 49–52
　diet. See Diet.
　handicapped. See Cerebral palsy; Heart disease;
　　and other illnesses.
　mouth hygiene,　38–41, 49–52
　safety education,　62
　self oral hygiene,　40
　x-ray examination,　124–125
Chocolate,　111
Chocolate milk,　110
Cleft lip,　7
Cleft palate,　7, 22
Cold sores,　21
Cosmetic dentistry,　59, 60–61
Council on Dental Therapeutics (American Dental
　　Association),　40

D

Dental floss,　52, 106
Dental health, diet relation,　109–113
Dental hygiene
　for children,　49
　for infants,　18, 19, 38–40
　for teenagers,　49–52
Dentin,　73–74
Dentistry
　cosmetic,　59, 60–61
　defensive,　2, 139
　of the future,　140
　interceptive,　140
　preventive,　137–139
　key tools in,　139
Dentists. See also Orthodontists; Periodontists.
　choosing,　115–117
　evaluating,　115, 117–118
　first visit to,　118–119
　frequency of visits to,　124
　pediatric,　116–117
　personality,　117
　respect for children,　119
　visit procedures,　119–123

Diet,　6, 7
　for adolescents,　65
　dental health relation,　109–113
　in pregnancy,　6, 7
　See also Food.
Disabilities,　22–23
Disclosing tablets,　92–93
Drooling,　31–32

E

Emergency treatment
　fractured tooth,　59
　knocked out tooth,　58–59
　toothache,　75
Enamel,　72–73
　demineralization,　103
　mineralization,　102, 103
Epstein's pearls,　9
Eruption cysts,　9

F

Falls,　58–59, 62
Fear,　120
Fetus, teeth of,　5, 6, 8
Fingernail biting,　45
First teeth. See Primary teeth.
Flossing,　52, 88–89
Fluoride
　cost of use,　99
　described,　97, 101
　endorsement of use,　99
　for infants,　10–11
　Kingston-Newburgh Study,　98–99
　misconceptions concerning,　100
　in mouthrinses,　40, 50, 90, 106
　reservoir,　78, 102–107
　safety of,　99
　supplements,　11, 94, 103–107
　systemic,　103–104
　in toothpastes,　40, 51, 91, 106
　topical,　40, 91, 94, 105–106
　vitamins with,　11
Fluorosis,　98, 104–105
Food. See also Diet.
　anti-cavity,　110, 111, 113
　bacteria and,　78, 110–111
　carbohydrates and cavities,　83, 110
　oral retention,　111, 112

snacks,   65, 96, 110–113, 139
soft vs hard,   20–21
Foreign objects,   47
Frenectomy,   34–35
Frenum,   34–35

G

Gingiva. *See* Gums.
Gingivitis,   84
Gum boil,   75
Gums,   76
    bleeding,   20, 64, 77
    pads, cleaning,   18–20, 31
    plaque and,   18, 19
    swollen,   6

H

Habits. *See also* specific habits, eg, Lip biting; thumb
        sucking, etc
    bad,   42–48, 131
    breaking of,   43, 47–48
    interceptive dentistry and,   129–131
    malocclusions and,   13, 42
    tooth position and,   13–14, 20–21, 42–48
Halitosis. *See* Bad breath.
Heart disease,   23
Hemophilia,   23
Herpes,   21

I

Illness
    childhood,   11, 12
    during pregnancy,   8
Implantation of teeth. *See* Primary teeth,
        implantation; Teeth, implantation.
Incisors, first appearance, 25–26, 28–29, 30–31
Infants
    cavities,   10
    dental hygiene for,   18–20
    feeding,   14–17
    fluoride for,   10–11
    soft vs hard food,   20–21
Infections
    control of transmission,   123
    during pregnancy,   8

of the mouth,   21, 75
Interdental devices,   91

J

Jawbone,   76

L

Lip biting,   43–44, 46

M

Malocclusion,   129
    caused by bad habits,   13, 14
    prevention,   13, 14, 129–131
    problems resulting from,   129
Mamelons,   34, 35
Mental retardation,   23
Milk,   15, 16, 110
    chocolate,   110
Milk teeth. *See* Primary teeth.
Minerals,   6
Molars
    first appearance,   27, 28–29, 30
    sealants for,   41
    six-year,   27, 33, 55
    surfaces,   6
Moniliasis. *See* Thrush.
Mouth
    bacteria,   10, 77, 78–79
    at birth,   8, 9
    examination,   39, 67–70
    hygiene,   18–20, 38–41, 81–94, 136
    infections,   21, 75
Mouth guards,   57, 62
Mouthrinses,   40, 50, 90, 106
    fluoride,   40, 50, 90, 106
Mouthwashes,   40, 50, 90

N

Nursing,   14
    bottle feeding,   14–17
    breast feeding,   14–15
Nutrition. *See* Diet; Food

O

Orthodontic appliances
    fixed vs removable,   135–136
Orthodontic treatment
    cost of,   134–135
    early,   132
    exercises,   131
    for improved appearance,   127–128
    lack of pain in,   135
    length of,   134
    medical reasons for,   128
    need for,   127–128
    oral hygiene during,   136
Orthodontics
    how it works,   132
    preventive,   129–131
Orthodontists, choosing, 132–134

P

Pacifiers,   12–13, 47
    substitutes for,   47
Parents
    fear of dentist,   120
    in treatment room,   121
Pediatric dentists. *See* Dentists, pediatric.
Pediatricians,   122
Pellicle. *See* Stains, black.
Periodontal ligament,   76
Periodontists,   35
Permanent teeth. *See* Teeth.
Phosphorus,   6
Plaque,   82–83
    bacteria and,   84–85
    control,   18–19, 84, 85–96
    decay and,   18, 83–84
    periodontal disease and,   84
    See also Mouth, hygiene; Teeth, cleaning
Pregnancy
    baby's teeth and,   6
    diet during,   6, 7
    infections during,   8
    tetracycline during,   8
    x-rays during,   8
Primary teeth
    cleaning,   18–20, 38–40
    color,   34
    crooked,   33
    decay,   10–11, 15–17
    development,   5–6, 28–29, 36–37, 71–72
    discolored,   26, 34
    effects on permanent teeth,   33, 58
    enamel defects,   26
    examination of,   39
    extra,   26–27
    first appearance. *See* Teething.
    function of,   32
    importance of,   32
    injuries and trauma,   33, 56, 58–59
    life cycle,   28–29
    loose,   55–56
    loss of,   33, 55–56
    problems with,   33
    reimplantation,   58–59
    retained too long,   130–131
    spaces between,   35
    structure,   33, 71–74
    supporting structures,   73, 76
    too few,   26
Pulp,   74

R

Retainers,   135

S

Saliva,   31–32, 77–78
Sealants,   41, 94–95
Smoking,   64
Snacks.   *See* Foods.
Space maintainers,   33, 130
Spaces,   35
Speech, teeth and,   48–49
Sports,   62
Stains
    black,   52, 53–54
    Colorado brown. *See* Fluorosis.
    orange,   52, 54
    green,   52, 53
    tetracycline,   8, 12, 52–53
Starches, cooked,   96, 110
Sucking,   5, 12–14
    See also Thumb sucking.
Sugars,   96, 110

T

Tartar,   76

Teenager
    bad breath,   64
    bleeding gums,   64
    bulimia,   66
    caries incidence,   139
    dental hygiene for,   63–66
    dentists and,   63
    diet,   65
    orthodontics for,   64
    smoking and,   64
    wisdom teeth,   65
Teeth. *See also* Canines; Incisors; Molars; Wisdom
        teeth.
    boys' vs girls',   26
    cleaning,   20, 38–40, 49–52
        See also Flossing; Toothbrushing.
    contouring,   95
    crooked,   33
    crowns of,   33, 72, 73
    decay. *See* Cavities.
    development,   5–6, 28–29, 36–37, 71–72
    effects of primary teeth on,   33, 58
    environment of,   76
    eruption,   5, 25–31
    fetal,   9
    first appearance,   25–31
    fractured,   58–59, 60
    injuries and trauma,   56, 58–59
    life cycle,   28–29
    occlusion,   55, 128–129
    position-habit relations,   13, 14, 20, 42
    primary. *See* Primary teeth.
    problems with,   33
    reimplantation,   58–59
    roots,   72, 76
        formation of,   5
    spaces between,   35
    speech and,   48–49
    stained. *See* Stains.
    structure,   71–74
    supporting structures,   73, 76
    surface of,   55, 94–95
    wisdom. *See* Wisdom teeth.
Teething,   10, 25, 30–31
    drooling and,   31–32
Tetracycline
    during pregnancy,   8
    stains,   8, 12, 52–53

Thrush,   21
Thumb sucking,   5, 46–47, 48
Tongue thrusting,   44, 46
Tongue tie,   22
Toothache
    emergency treatment,   75
    types,   75
Toothbrushes,   39–40, 49–50, 89–90
    electric,   50, 90
Toothbrushing,   39–40
    "Buddy system,"   93–94
    techniques,   85–87
Tooth Fairy,   56
Tooth grinding,   45–46
Toothpastes,   39, 40, 51, 91–92, 93, 106
    for children,   39, 40, 51, 91–92
    fluoride,   51, 91, 106

U

US Centers for Disease Control,   123
US Public Health Service,   98, 99

V

Vitamins, with fluoride,   11

W

Water-irrigating devices,   51–52, 65
Water Pik®,   51
Wisdom teeth,   65

X

X-rays
    during pregnancy,   8
    examinations,   124–125